Vision for the Future

Meeting the Challenge of Sight Loss

of related interest

Approaches to Case Management for People with Disabilities
Doria Pilling
ISBN 1 85302 099 0

How to Get Equipment for Disability (2nd edition)
Compiled by Michael Mandelstam
ISBN 1 85302 128 8

Managing Disability at Work
Improving Practice in Organisations
Brenda Smith, Margery Povall and Michael Floyd
ISBN 1 85302 123 7

The Psychology of Ageing
An Introduction
Ian Stuart-Hamilton
ISBN 1 85302 063 X

Children with Special Needs
Assessment, Law and Practice –
Caught in the Act
Harry Chasty and John Friel
ISBN 1 85302 096 6

Vision for the Future

Meeting the Challenge of Sight Loss

Maria C. Conyers

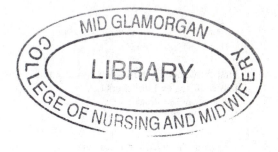

Jesssica Kingsley Publishers
London and Philadelphia

First published in the United Kingdom in 1992 by
Jessica Kingsley Publishers Ltd
118 Pentonville Road
London N1 9JB

Copyright © 1992 Maria Conyers

British Library Cataloguing in Publication Data
Conyers, Maria
Vision for the Future: Meeting the
Challenge of Sight Loss
I. Title
617.7

ISBN 1-85302-110-5

Printed and Bound in Great Britain by
Bookcraft Ltd., Avon

31·10·96

To my husband, Michael, and daughter,
Cassandra, with love

Acknowledgements

A debt of personal gratitude is owed to numerous individuals and organisations who were supportive of the concept of this study, not least my employing Authority at that time, and medical colleagues. It is not feasible to list all those numerous colleagues and friends who have generously given of their time, both their personal and professional experience, to share ideas, crystallise aims, generally offering constructive comment and moral support along the way.

Thanks are extended to both the local authority specialist visual impairment teams for their tremendous enthusiasm and commitment. Without the support and insight of the teams and their managers, together with the courage of the clients themselves, this study would not have been possible.

A particular debt of gratitude is owed to Jacqueline Blanchard of the London Hospital Bereavement Service for her unflagging and constant wisdom, insight and practical support throughout the early stages of this study.

Amongst others, Pat Schoffield, Celia Tickner, Andrea Stoltmeir made various helpful suggestions concerning the design and practical implementation of the interview; as did also Susan Le Poidivin and others. Their combined comments were much appreciated and contributed to the overall effectiveness and outcome of this project.

Others to be thanked are Caroline Wilkinson together with Barbara Wade who were responsible for the computer analysis. Their tolerance and humorous guidance concerning my tentative steps into the world of computers was much appreciated.

Heartfelt thanks are extended to Professor Eric Sainsbury and David Phillips of Sheffield University who have jointly shared their considerable, individual specialist experience in guiding the writing of this book.

I am appreciative of the assistance given by the Kings Fund who initially financed the study.

Lynn Crichton and Diane Cass painstakingly typed the many drafts of this book, to them I offer special thanks.

It would be invidious to try and name particular individuals, as without the enormous goodwill and generosity of so many people this study would never have come to fruition.

Maria C. Conyers
July 1991

Special Notes

Terminology

1. It will be noted that when talking of the visually impaired collectively, both the terms of 'patient' and 'client' are used in the text. This seems realistic because when someone is losing sight they enter the hospital system and are denoted as patients. As the career in disability unfolds and they have contact with social workers, they tend to be known as clients. At the end of the day, whatever they are termed, we must remember that each disabled individual remains uniquely themselves—a person in their own right.

2. 'Traumatic loss' of sight refers to the period from onset, within days or weeks, up to six months.

3. 'Degenerative loss' of sight refers to onset from six months up to several years.

4. 'Blind' and/or 'partial sight' refers to classification for registration purposes.

Contents

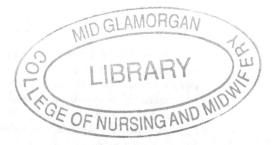

Acknowledgements   6

Special notes   6

Foreword   9

1. Early days: Background and Initiation of the Study   11

Introduction/Interviewing patients/Profile of participating local authorities

2. Some Thoughts on Losing Sight: Literature Survey   22

General understanding of loss of sight/The role of the Ophthalmologist/Patients' response to registration as visually impaired

3. The Career Begins: Awareness of Sight Loss   28

Introduction/The General Practitioner

4. The Career Progresses: Contact With the Opthalmologist   34

Introduction/Seeing the Ophthalmologist and explanation of diagnosis/ Did the Ophthalmologist help prepare 'patients' for sight loss?/The doctor/patient relationship and potential for change/Conclusions/Recommendations

5. Registration: A Point of No Return'?   45

Introduction/Patients' feelings and perceptions concerning registration/Acute psycho-social distress/Stigmatisation/ Negative denial response/Resignation/Preparation for registration/Perceived advantages and disadvantages of registration/The administration of the registration process

6. 'What Does the Future Hold for Me Now'? Evaluation of
   Patients' Psycho-social Response to Loss of Vision   66

   Introduction/Do we become what we think we are?/Case
   examples and alternatives for practice/The psychological
   and social reaction to loss of sight/Practical adjustment/
   Physical health/Worry, anxiety, emotional pain, puzzlement/
   Denial, despair, anger, bitterness, refusal to accept/
   Self-image/Relationships with others/Negative changes in
   Social relationships/Conclusions

7. Counselling and What it Means to Clients   87

   Introduction/'Counselling'—The case presentation of
   'Mary'/The case presentation of Lottie/Who should provide
   a counselling service?/Conclusions and recommendations

8. New Roads Lie Ahead: Rehabilitation After Care Services   106

   Introduction/How patients managed before assistance was provided/The
   types of help offered and perceived/Thoughts
   on who most helped clients work through feelings about loss
   of sight/Did rehabilitation change perceptions about visual
   impairment?/Summary

9. Arriving and Feeling Comfortable with Ourselves:
   The Question of Adjustment   119

10. Major Recommendations   126

Appendix   128

Bibliography   136

Index   138

Foreword

This work draws upon a four year investigation co-ordinated by the author, exploring how individuals and their families have been affected by, and how they cope with, the experience of sight loss; whether onset is gradual (degenerative) or sudden (traumatic) partial or total loss of sight. In short, to consider the patients' 'career in disability' from a social, emotional and psychological view-point. The study draws on their perceptions of these experiences from the onset of awareness of visual impairment, through registration, rehabilitation and beyond. By eliciting patients' views about the service they received, from their general practitioner, ophthalmologist and social services departments, the aim is to consider what impact diagnosis and prognosis has on the patient, and to explore whether the manner in which bad news is broken may ultimately affect healthy adjustment to loss of sight. Questioning the definitions of such terms as adjustment and acceptance, and what qualitatively makes for a healthier emotional and psychological response to loss of sight, was also the intention of this study.

Loss of vision, of any degree, is clearly a subjective, personal, internal experience calling potentially for major life changes. Loss of vision impinges on every facet of daily living affecting self-image, social relationships, status, practical 'taken for granted' capabilities and skills, potentially undermining confidence and previously established self-perceptions and patterns of behaviour, lifestyle, occupation, etc. How one responds to this type of crisis, or any form of disability or illness, originates in previous experiences of losses and the manner in which these challenges have been met.

The degree of preparation for sight loss is now thought to be significant; how much warning an individual needs in order to prepare both practically and emotionally for the deterioration of sight loss is a factor of which all health care professionals need to be aware. However, the results from this investigation suggest that there is a tendency for all those involved in the care of patients to give insufficient importance to the need for emotional and psychological preparation.

The cornerstone of this study was the assumption that patients cannot begin to adjust unless they know what it is they have to potentially face and adjust to. In working through this insight at the patients' own pace they need to be helped to tolerate what cannot be changed and to alter what can be altered.

The evidence from this study suggests that a major area of patients' needs, if not actually overlooked, is not being met, and that their greatest difficulty lies in intellectual, psychological and emotional resolution.

From the evidence of the patients interviewed concerning their relationships with members of the multi-disciplinary team, it is suggested that the ophthalmologist may not necessarily be the most appropriate or only member of the team to break bad news concerning sight loss. The merits of multi-disciplinary training in counselling for the visually impaired is considered, along with a discussion of the conflicts between cost effectiveness of counselling, resource allocation and policy decisions about service provision.

The question of ethics and morality in interviewing patients was one debated at length. However, patients' qualitative insights have a crucial place in social work investigation with its holistic connotations. One of the aims was to communicate with the medical profession in its own language.

With hindsight it is acknowledged that the content and statistics could have legitimately formed the basis of further work. It is hoped, nevertheless, that the content of this book will enlighten, provoke and stimulate.

Chapter 1

Early Days
Background and Initiation of the Study

Introduction

In attempting to set up and provide a social work service in a busy and hard pressed ophthalmology out-patient department, several issues relating to patient care seemed to call for further exploration.

There were apparent divisions and what appeared to be mutually exclusive interests of medical, nursing personnel and local authority social workers. These professions seemed to have little more than a cursory, superficial understanding of the pressures, constraints and potentialities of the others' professional role. Somewhere, our patients were caught in the centre of this confusion. It appeared there was a risk of well-intentioned professionals neatly packaging or categorizing patients' needs. In this way, the complexity of patients' social and emotional response to loss of sight seemed in danger of being dissipated, distorted, or worse perhaps, overlooked. It seemed important to provide feed-back about the internal upheaval that loss of sight may provoke; and in so doing to highlight patients' wider psychological needs, outside of their six monthly or annual clinic appointment or statutory contact following registration with their social services department.

Another matter, which is discussed in greater detail elsewhere in this book, is that prior to the initiation of the study it was necessary to clarify understanding on the ways in which medical staff deal with the unavoidable feelings of failure in treating patients whose sight loss cannot be reversed or halted. Most professionals can find it difficult to know how to manage, or cope with situations where there are no ideal solutions to major problems. For the patient who is losing or who has lost sight, it may appear that medicine has failed. Patients generally tend to ascribe considerable therapeutic powers to their doctors and assume that medicine can or should alleviate their problem in some way. This situation can be very problematic for doctors and other carers who have to find ways of coping with their own sense of hurt, disappointment and failure when treating patients whose sight loss cannot be reversed or halted. One way of doing so is adoption of what the psychoanalysts have called denial; namely, an unconscious tendency to underplay the seriousness of the situation. This mechanism may be found both in the patients faced with the tragic outcome and in those who care for them—their professional helpers, their families—so there is sometimes a kind of collusion maintaining the phenomenon of denial, but with the inevitable risk that the subsequent reality becomes even harder to bear, especially for the patients when they eventually become aware of the permanency or irreversibility of sight loss.

This type of denial might be expressed in the unconscious delaying of registration involving delayed completion of BD8 forms (which admits patients to the Register of Visually Impaired People in Great Britain) or prevarication about which category patients should be registered under, e.g. partially sighted or blind. Discussions with other colleagues suggested that such a process of delay, if detectable, tends to be rationalized as breaking the patients in gently, shielding them from the painful realisation of sight loss. This is dealt with in Chapter 6. Sometimes it is suggested that a patient will not cope with the truth, and that therefore they should not be given a clear or full prognosis.

The growing feeling that patients very often leave out- patients clinics either unaware that they have been registered as visually impaired, or fail to understand the implications of registration, suggested the need for a detailed investigation looking at the three steps culminating in registration as visually impaired, i.e. diagnosis/pre-registration; registration as visually impaired (blind/partially-sighted); and post-registration, after-care and rehabilitation.

Another aim was to consider whether resource allocation, staffing levels and training might impinge on, if not effectively alter, the nature of the doctor/patient or social worker/client relationships. This type of analysis can be potentially problematic.

A central assertion of the study was that insufficient counselling and emotional support is available to the visually impaired. It was felt that the reasons for this lack of particular assistance were various and complex, bound up in the relationships and expectations between patients and the professionals involved with their care. Therefore, an ensuing and underpinning aim of this project was that the study should constitute more than an exploratory document, but should seek to extend its boundaries; highlighting not only possible shortfalls in service delivery and care, but also to underline the positive areas for potential development, improvement and growth. Thus, it was felt desirable that a diagnostic component of the study should point the way to complimentary and alternative measures in the treatment and care of the visually impaired and their families.

By asking patients to first recall their experience as consumers, i.e. being on the receiving end of medical and social work assistance, and second to evaluate the service they were offered, the intention was to provide much-needed information for all professionals involved with the management and care of the visually impaired. It was felt desirable that such information should be made widely available to interested professionals, in order that current organisation of individual professional practice and multi-disciplinary collaboration and service delivery be reviewed.

What must be acknowledged from the outset is that first, whilst this investigation was drawn out of a lengthy study spanning two years and involving two London boroughs, no claims are made as to the findings being applicable to other geographical areas. Because of the nature of the investigation, statistical testing of the representative nature of the work was not possible. Therefore no statistical conclusions are drawn from the results of the study. Rather the aim and desire is to present cumulative reflection and insight derived from clinical experience of counselling and from the patients interviewed in this study. Furthermore, literature which has been pertinent to further understanding about loss of vision will be considered. This book is intended as a practical handbook for any professional who has contact with people losing their sight. Furthermore, this book could be helpful for people losing sight, their families or loved ones, as a reference source or to enlighten their experience.

Readers should realise that this work was carried out in addition to the author's professional commitment as a social worker. This was also true for the colleagues who volunteered to act as interviewers. All had professional knowledge and some had personal experience of visual impairment. Prior to the initiation of the study there was liaison with senior social services and medical nursing personnel, to discuss the need for such a study. This was especially important as little or no additional time could be allocated as at the outset financial support was uncertain. It was an unequivocal reality that the setting up of the project would depend largely on the goodwill and commitment of all staff involved. These factors, it was accepted, would have general implications, but particularly for the recruitment and inclusion of the participating authorities. The project therefore had to be limited in scope.

The project was divided into three sections:

1. Planning, training and pilot study.
2. The interviewing of patients.
3. Consideration of findings, completion of interim paper and book.

In total, nine inner London and suburban authorities were approached who were thought to be likely candidates on the basis of their varied health and welfare provision and the different ratios of specialist workers to the visually impaired population. Initially three local authorities within the Greater London area sought to be included. One withdrew in the early stages for the same reason that other authorities had cited, namely, staff shortages and pressure on existing services to meet statutory demands. Although no significant differences were found between the participating boroughs in respect of patients' needs and experiences, the two remaining authorities were thought to be quite different in character and orientation of philosophy for service provision. Furthermore, a main purpose of the project was to explore the inner life and experience of the disabled person, which would have general relevance for the vast majority of visually impaired people. It is not the intention to concentrate excessively on the different demographic features or aspects such as client/staff ratio which were found to be of minimal importance, and implications of which could be construed as implying a political judgment.

The content and structure of the interview procedure was evolved following discussion with many colleagues, including the research departments within respective authorities, specialist workers, some of whom were visually impaired themselves, and other interested professionals. The design was continually refined both prior to and following the pilot study. The interview was divided into the three phases of the visually impaired person's career in disability: diagnosis and pre-registration; registration; rehabilitation and after-care. An additional personality assessment sought to explore the total (holistic) experience of patients, considering their psychological, emotional and social responses and pre-dispositions at three stages, namely:

a) before loss of sight occurred;

b) at time of loss; and

c) following loss of sight—currently when interviewed.
(Refer to Appendix 1 for interview format.)

It was decided early on that, because of the emotive and searching nature of the interview, it would not be in the clients' best interests to use external professional interviewing teams who would have no experience of visual impairment or even perhaps of this type of interview (with counselling undertones). The interviewing teams therefore comprised of experienced specialist social workers in visual impairment who were trained in the techniques necessary for the study. Training was spread over 14 hours and comprised role play interview technique, the identification of possible problems arising and appropriate responses. Attention was also paid to particular issues within the interview which the interviewers feared they would find difficult: for example, raising the issue of suicide or discussion about intimate relationships. Interviewers were also instructed to report patients' verbatim responses to the open-ended qualitative questions. Within both authorities, workers interviewed each others' clients rather than their own; interviewers were instructed not to interview any person who was previously known to them. The hope was in this way, to optimise information gathering whilst retaining an understanding style of interviewing. Initially regular on- going fortnightly supervision was given to the teams to elicit any difficulties or questions that arose from the interviewing of patients. Counselling was available for patients, if it was felt necessary, following the study interview. (The case of Mary, which is presented in Chapter 7, is an example.) The author was available to provide informal supervision of specific cases, and the implications of these referrals were also discussed at the group meetings.

A small pilot study was conducted, on a random selection of 20 patients drawn from each authority and evaluated as being suitable for inclusion in the study because of age, gender, and origin of loss. The interview design was accordingly adjusted as the experience gained in this phase was used to complement the training of interviewers.

Interviewing of patients

Patients were contacted by letter outlining the reason for the study and requesting their permission for inclusion in the project. An appointment was made and people were visited either in their own home or, if requested by them, on neutral territory such as a local day centre or agreed office. Wherever possible patients were interviewed on their own. It was noted that some spouses/families appeared to exert strong pressure on patients to allow them to be present. This was particularly prevalent amongst the elderly.

The interviews lasted on average for between one and two hours. In the case of the elderly, where it was felt appropriate, interviews were sometimes spread over two sessions. Interpreters were used for those where English was not the language of origin, though this only applied to seven people within the group. Note was made of additional handicaps, with particular reference to disabilities which might significantly affect the interview responses, such as deafness or hard of hearing. We were also aware that additional physical handicap might colour patients' perceptions of visual impairment and its long term effects. Interviewers were encouraged to make a separate record of any significant factors arising from the interview which was not previously included in the interview.

Information from the closed and multi-choice questions were analyzed on computer. The study was concerned primarily to explore patients' emotional and psychological responses to loss of sight. One of the study's aims was to value the subtle nuances of patients' perceptions and experiences, despite inherent difficulties of interpretation. However, it was considered to be desirable and necessary to develop a sense of self-criticism to strive for high standards. It seems appropriate to put on record the possible shortcomings and limitations of the study and to respond to them.

First, it is accepted that there is a negative bias in the construction of questions within the interview questionnaire. There was, however, a philosophy and purpose underlying such a design, particularly in the holistic section. The intention was to identify particular areas of significant difficulty. In the interview structure questions were designed to also focus on dimensions of human response. Thus, the intellectual, emotional and behavioural dimensions explored touched necessarily on intimate and highly sensitive issues such as sexuality, suicide, and addictive tendencies. From clinical experience of patients who are working through or facing severe irreversible disablement (including visual impairment) or bereavement, it has been noted that the defence mechanism of denial is frequently unconsciously employed. This tendency linked to patients' inhibition to openly admit having powerful negative feelings could, it was believed, block patients' ability to answer questions honestly. Therefore, in an attempt to implicitly give patients permission to own and ventilate their feelings, particularly concerning social taboos, we asked if certain statements were common to their experiences of life and loss of sight, before, during, or following loss. In this way patients then had the opportunity to refute or agree with the statements. These statements were compiled and derived from the most common sentiments and statements made by numerous patients on whom clinical records had previously been kept. They were felt to be indicative of the most frequent range of responses to visual loss. Patients were asked, for example, whether they had thought of taking their own life and, if so, whether they had ever made a suicide attempt. In the case of one lady, this question allowed her to acknowledge for the first time, unknown to her family and the rehabilitation officer, that these matters were very powerful difficulties for her. She had covered up her feelings successfully for a long time and arguably might never have disclosed either her suicidal urges or her misconstrued previous attempts. Though this was a dramatic disclosure for this patient, it opened the way to the counselling help she needed, because the secrecy she had employed to hide her suicidal urges was achieved at a price, becoming increasingly difficult to suppress and emotionally turbulent for her. It appeared that the interview had been cathartic, allowing her to disclose these pressures and to begin to explore her needs and what assistance was available.

Second, the group was not demographically representative, but rather constituted the whole population of newly registered people in two authorities in one year. As previously mentioned, the exploration of the clients' inner lives, in terms of general trends, may have relevance to the whole of the visually impaired population, but this is far from conclusive. Those patients in employment, the under-40s group, and ethnic minorities were too small a number to be representative from which to draw firm conclusions.

The third area of difficulty in such an investigation is the use and potential abuse of value laden and inherently subjective concepts, such as the evaluation of adequacy or sympathy. Such words mean different things to different people. The author has attempted to overcome this problem by the inclusion of closed questions, multi-choice answers, complemented by patients' individual reflective statements. Throughout the text there will be an elaboration of these themes as appropriate.

Profile of participating local authorities

The ethics of the project were examined at every stage. One of the primary objectives of this study was to sensitively explore clients' emotional responses and needs following loss of sight. It was therefore essential that, as far as possible, this concern should extend to the interviewing of patients. Careful consideration was given, therefore, to the selection of patients for the study. It was decided to include only those who had been registered with local authority social services departments as visually impaired (blind or partially sighted) for at least six months, but not exceeding two years. All patients who had been registered between the 1st January and 31st December 1984 were included. The philosophy behind this decision was that while patients' experiences and memories might still be clear enough for the purposes of the study, their recollections would not be too immediately distressing during interview. As noted earlier, follow-up professional counselling was made available to anyone who requested help either as a consequence of the interview—stirring painful memories—or as a general result of visual impairment. The total group for the study from the participating authorities was 122. Children under 18 years old were excluded from the study on two grounds: first, that the needs and services available to children differ quantitatively and generally from those of the adult population; and second, that the majority of visually impaired people originate from the adult population.

Eighteen further patients were excluded on the basis of psychiatric unsuitability or gross medical incapacitation. In the case of one elderly woman who was profoundly deaf and had gross communication problems, it was felt unethical to burden her with an interview. These omissions do not suggest that the experiences of those excluded had nothing to offer, but rather reflect concern to maintain the rights of the vulnerable patients.

Authority 'A'

Authority 'A' is situated within an industrialized urban city area with all the problems and characteristics commonly associated with such environments. The total borough population is in the region of 148,700, of which 25,000 are aged between 60 and 85 years of age. At the time, there were approximately 780 visually handicapped inhabitants who were registered. The rate of non-registered referrals made to the centrally based specialist team within the borough is about equal to those who are registered. The specialist team responded to approximately 80 to 100 referrals for both blind and partially sighted people.

The specialist team which provided the service across the borough was headed by a team leader and comprised two specialist workers and technical officers with access to external borough mobility training. The specialist team was sub-divided into two smaller teams catering for the needs of the visually or hearing impaired population.

The team took referrals from any source, not just people eligible to be registered as visually impaired. The aim was that all new referrals received a visit by a technical officer for assessment usually within one to two months.

The team's priorities, unless otherwise requested, usually encompassed people of working age, the elderly blind living alone or with relatives, the elderly blind in residential care or elderly partially sighted people living alone. Consideration was also given to elderly partially sighted within the community.

The team's rehabilitation programme encompassed teaching daily living skills provided in the patient's home, and residential courses funded by social services departments. Such rehabilitation might include communication skills, typing, braille, moon (again taught in patient's home) and mobility training outdoors, in which case a sessional mobility officer might be used with concentration given to learning routes to work, day centres, etc. Orientation and support is also offered to patients and staff within the residential care setting, comprising Local Authority, private and voluntary Part III 'Residential care for the elderly'.

The philosophy of the specialist team was to provide services, counselling and training to all affected individuals and family, focusing on aspects of rehabilitation, employment, leisure activities and information giving, with regular follow-up support both pre- and post-registration. The team aimed to contact every client at least once a year.

It was noted in Authority 'A' that although there was some contact with specialist hospital social workers, most of the work was carried out by generic based social workers often in conjunction with technical officers within the borough.

The ophthalmology service located within a major teaching hospital had spasmodic and infrequent face-to-face contact with the specialist team. There appeared to be some difficulty in setting up workable channels of communication. The ethos of the specialist team was to maintain and enhance the level of independence for their visually impaired clients.[1]

Authority 'B'

Authority 'B' is one of the largest inner London boroughs with a population of around 240,000, and experienced the complete range of urban problems.

At the time of the study there were over 1000 people in the borough who are registered blind or partially sighted. At least 95 percent of those registered were over 60 years old, often with other physical disabilities.

Each year the centrally based Visual Impairment Specialist Team assesses approximately 1040 people newly registered blind or partially sighted and processes an even larger number of referrals. The specialist team comprised of a team manager, senior social worker, social worker, social welfare officer, senior rehabilitation or mobility officer, rehabilitation officer (activities), rehabilitation officer (mobility), sessional rehabilitation officer and a team clerk.

---

[1] Information supplied by Ms P Schofield, Team Manager, Visual Impairment Specialist Services Team.

The pre- and post-registration service provided by the team included assessment, counselling, advice, information, rehabilitation and special equipment. Work was undertaken with all ages, both individually and in groups, within peoples' homes, work places, schools, or at a rehabilitation flat.

The team's philosophy was to enable visually impaired people to maintain independence by maximizing their potential whatever the circumstances.

Two major ophthalmic referral units were based within the Authority's catchment area; one was a London teaching hospital and the other, as previously stated, was Moorfields.[2]

The group

Overall it was noted that within the group the female population was larger than the male group: 71 female patients as against 33 males. There does appear to be an epidemiological trend in western cultures of women living longer than men and at the older end of the age scales for the female population to predominate, though no strong contentions are made in the case of this study.

English was the language of origin or defined first language for the majority of the group. It is perhaps surprising that only six patients reported English as being their second language, particularly when we consider that both participating authorities have substantial ethnic populations. Equally puzzling was the fact that for just under a quarter of the group, this information was either not forthcoming from the patients themselves or was not otherwise available for our records.

The biggest religious denomination represented amongst the interviewees, just under two-thirds, were Protestant, defining themselves Church of England, with 17 Roman Catholic patients forming the second largest religious group. There were no patients of Muslim, Hindu or Jewish faith, which links with the small number of ethnic groups within the study. However, nine patients, while specifying allegiance to other religious beliefs, declined to elaborate, with a further 13 patients giving no answer.

Only three people from the group were in employment at the time of the interview. In terms of socio-economic status, for which patients were asked to rate themselves, the biggest single group, over one-third of the total, described themselves as manual or unskilled workers. About another third, 32, defined themselves as having been in skilled or semi-skilled trades. Although 20 were unable to answer, it was also noted that the smallest group, 16 patients, ranked themselves as being professional or white collar workers.

---

[2] Information supplied by Mr Peter Davies-Finley, Team Manager, Visual Impairment Specialist Services Team.

The group was too small to establish any correlation between type or rank of occupation with incidence of sight loss, nor was it one of the aims, but perhaps it would constitute further interesting research.

The extent of sight loss within the group was fairly evenly spread, with 54 percent being registered blind and 46 percent partially sighted. Perhaps not so surprisingly, degenerative or gradual loss of sight was the largest origin of loss, 7 percent suffering traumatic sight loss. As will be seen later in this book, many factors may account for this, such as advances in surgical reconstructive technology avoiding the devastation of what may have formerly constituted traumatic visual impairment.

Although nine patients reported secondary disabilities other than visual impairment, undoubtedly the largest additional handicap was that of hearing disability, with over a quarter experiencing some difficulty in this area.

It is of interest to note that both the patients and the interviewers undertook parallel journeys. The intention of the study was to log clients' careers in disability, their thoughts, feelings and responses to the massive life change that loss of sight entails. In undertaking this study, a journey of discovery was commenced. The journey for patients begins when they first become aware that there is something wrong with their vision. This book therefore outlines and examines patients' experiences in four main stages:

1. Contact with general practitioners.
2. The hospital experience and preliminary discussions about registration as visually impaired.
3. First contact with social services departments and rehabilitative services.
4. After-care and beyond.

During these phases patients' experiences are discussed along with the implications for practice and policy planning. Inherent in the discussion is the psychological and social management of patients as they pass through the health and welfare systems.

The latter chapters offer specific practical advice on the establishment of a multi-disciplinary counselling team. The case examples are offered in the hope that they will serve as a catalyst to further thinking and practice in caring for those who have failing vision. The practical advice offered in these chapters can be viewed as elementary tools to assist in the exploration and venting of disease in the very broadest sense. The musings in this text may be a bitter pill to swallow, or the advice may fall on stony ground. Others may feel that much that is said may contain little which is intrinsically new. The justification would be that what needs to be voiced and loses nothing by being freshly affirmed, is that the needs, feelings and rights of patients have to be of paramount importance.

Chapter 10 presents an overview of the study and concludes with major recommendations.

Summary of aims

1. To investigate wider psychological, emotional and social response to loss of sight.

2. To provide feed-back to medical and community personnel about the current service offered to patients, and their perception and evaluation of the care they received.

3. To explore the three phases of a career in disability: diagnosis, registration and aftercare.

4. To explore the nature of the relationship between doctor and patient and social worker during a two year period, encompassing the three phases above.

5. From the results and deliberations of the study, to provide a diagnostic commentary highlighting potential areas for improvement.

6. To postulate and outline complementary and alternative measures for the psychological management of patients.

7. To extrapolate main conclusions relevant to policy making and to the development of service procedures.

Chapter 2

Some Thoughts on Losing Sight
Literature Survey

When considering the needs of and services available to the visually handicapped population, it is helpful to reflect on the emotional responses, social
pressures, and practical everyday concerns that may affect them, and also
their families and friends. A review of relevant literature needs to reflect, as
far as possible, these same concerns. It is the author's intention that this
section should serve more as an appetizer used for comparison, providing
background insight for the reader. The boundaries of this project were
broadly placed and therefore any such study, realistically, can only point the
motivated reader in the right direction. Additional references will be made
to other contributors throughout the text, particularly where specific comments or comparisons are felt to be helpful.

General understanding of sight loss

There are several papers exploring reactions to specific causes of loss of sight,
such as Oehler-Giarrantana & Fitzgerald (1980), while others detail the
emotional needs of a particular sub-group of the visually impaired population, such as the emotional reactions and fears of newly visually impaired
adolescents, for example Calek (1980) and Ollendick (1985). More person-
alised individual case studies, such as Hoehn-Saric (1981), have provided
more intimate anecdotal accounts. Direct comparison between these papers
and the present more general investigation is complex. Dunton's early study
of the newly blind in 1908 noted that reactive depression usually followed
awareness of non-reversible sight loss and that suicidal thoughts were
common. However, he concluded attempts at suicide were more rare. Witt-
kower and Davenport's (1946) survey of the war blinded (traumatic loss)
recorded similar responses and defined shock, disbelief (inability to accept
the fact of loss) and denial as commonplace. Cholden's (1950) extensive work
with the blind led him to analogize the emotional effect of irreversible
blindness for the patient to the death of a loved one, insofar as the patient
suffers the death of a sighted person within himself. He needs to work
through a period of grief and mourning towards 'healthy' resolution and
assimilation of the crisis. However, despite Cholden's many sensitive in-

sights there is a subtle but implicit assumption that this mourning process can be navigated, in most cases, with the passage of time.

It seems probable from the accounts of patients in this book, that whilst it may superficially appear that working through and adjustment to disability has taken place, with the outward resumption of daily and social living skills, there is the growing awareness that at a deeper level the work of mourning such loss may be at best extended through years, and for some may never entirely be given up.

The work of mourning disability may be viewed as an insidious tidal process. At times of external pressure, either from family relationships, financial hardship or lack of social status, the effect of mourning lost sight may be exacerbated, to diminish later once again.

Fitzgerald's survey (1970) of newly blinded patients concludes that shock, denial, anger and anxiety are essentially healthy responses (particularly in the early stages) to loss of sight. He found that for between 85 and 92 percent depression was the most common response, but noted that it is the prolongation of symptoms which ultimately constitutes a pathological grief reaction, not the initial reaction itself. Fitzgerald also concluded that forewarning of visual loss did not appear to significantly help the patient's adjustment. Fitzgerald did not pursue in depth the manner in which forewarning of sight loss was given to the patients in his study, or the bearing this might have on their long term adjustment. Furthermore, it was not in the scope of his study to compare or measure the affect of forewarning on practical adjustment as opposed to emotional well-being. Diamond & Ross (1945) suggested that the ability to accept finality of loss and the surrendering of false hopes is an early predictor of healthier adjustment to loss of sight. This raises speculation about the role of the ophthalmologist in breaking bad news (refer also to Chapter 4).

Other factors affecting levels of social and emotional adjustment were noted by Ash, Keegan and Greenough (1978a & b) in their study which considered the presence or otherwise of an additional physical handicap. For example, neuromuscular conditions co- existing with visual impairment suggested that poorer all round adjustment was more likely. Pre-existing personality traits such as shyness or excessive humility were also noted as adverse factors in adjustment, giving a higher preponderance of dependent psychological reactions, i.e. becoming excessively dependent on care givers. Not surprisingly, Schultz (1979) suggested that the family played a crucial part in the individual's adjustment to his/her visual disability. He cited four reactions with which the family may present:

Overprotection—which reinforces dependence and may therefore have some linkage with Ash's conclusions. Furthermore, Dr. Shaw's Survey commented that of the 19 local authorities participating in the review and analysis of rehabilitation service provision, 12 local authority social services departments cited overprotection of the visually

handicapped 'by parents or other family members' as being a significant factor determining whether or not, and to what extent, residential
rehabilitation is taken up by the affected person. In connection to the
concept of overprotection, it was noted in this study that frequently
other family members requested, and on occasion insisted, that they be
present during the study interview. This was particularly the case with
elderly participants, often even when the patient had stated they
wished to be interviewed alone.

Denial—generally defined as an inability to accept or take in the fact
(reality) of visual impairment. A detailed evaluation of the incidence
and types of denial thought to be present in relation to sight loss will
be given in Chapters 5 and 6.

Rejection by family members—There was little evidence of this latter trait.
In this book, findings suggest that 14 people felt family relationships
had changed for the better following loss of sight. On the other hand
only eight people felt family relationships had changed for the worse.
People spoke of feeling warmer, having got closer through the crisis of
coping with a disability. In some instances it was felt that having to ask
for assistance from family members had given the opportunity for
changed relationships. However, 36 patients in our investigation expressed fear about other people's (society's) rejection. As will be seen
in the latter chapters, there was genuine concern surrounding whether
or not people would feel stigmatised by their disability or, worse still,
patronized and pitied.

Acceptance—which is also listed by Adams, Pearlman and Sloan (1971)
as one of the three primary and most common responses to loss of sight,
may be said to have been achieved when the afflicted person could
tolerate and accept the changes that loss of sight had brought, feeling
relatively at ease with his/her self image; adapting behaviour to meet
these changes; formulating a life style which was defined as being
relatively anxiety free as far as it relates to the disability. It may be
argued that the term "acceptance" is overly and inappropriately used.
What is deemed as "acceptance" may vary widely from individual to
individual.

Lukoff and Whitman (1972) conclude from their research that the higher the
level of education, the more satisfactory was the level of adaptation. This
links with Ash's study where evidence suggested that good education and
high socio-economic status was found to be of benefit in overall adjustment
to visual loss. This was felt in part to be due to the fact that these people were
found to be less likely affected by the direct consequences of visual impairment, particularly in terms of employment, financial income, and sense of
status. Conversely, it was noted that the poorer and less educated the patient,
the more likely were problems in social and emotional adjustment. Lukoff's

and Ash's papers could have usefully been extended to consider whether the apparent correlation between high socio-economic status and education and satisfactory adaption to loss, was because people in these groups might have the necessary opportunities and communication skills to more effectively ventilate their emotional distress and obtain the required assistance. In the absence of such consideration, therefore, it may be necessary to hypothesize that deprived inner city areas would benefit from targeting rehabilitation and counselling resources, to meet the needs of the visually impaired in those areas.

The role of the ophthalmologist

It is a fundamental concern of this book to consider the central bearing that the relationship between ophthalmologist and patient can have on long term emotional and psychological adjustment to loss of sight. The author unreservedly agrees with Rakes and Reid's (1982) conclusions on the psychological management of loss of vision that:

> The ophthalmologist is in the unique position to positively influence the lives of these individuals (patients) providing that he or she is interested and available and has the confidence, reassurance and caring that can help blind patients remain active well adjusted members of society.

Valid though such sentiments are, sadly they would appear to be an ideal which is yet to be attained. The impressions gathered in this book from the patients interviewed was that more time for discussion and sharing of concerns would have been welcomed.

Greenblatt's research (1986) concerning ophthalmologist/patient interactions amongst 410 practising ophthalmologists in one American state, illustrated that patients with less severe defects (acuity range 20/20 but better than 20/200) seemed to receive less discussion about diagnosis and prognosis or referral for rehabilitation services. All practitioners intimated that discussions about diagnosis and prognosis were more likely to be initiated where visual acuity was 20/200 or less. She concluded that, 'at less severe levels of impairment however, when the final level of impairment has not been reached, ophthalmologists seemed to avoid informing patients of their diagnosis.' (1986) Reluctance on the part of ophthalmologists to come clean about the expected degree of deterioration denies the disabled patient the opportunity to make adequate preparation for the future. Such anticipatory preparation should ideally be both practical and emotional. The benefits of honest disclosure of prognosis and the facilitation of preparedness will be considered in depth in Chapters 4 and 6.

Furthermore, it was noted that ophthalmologists were an isolated profession, liaising very infrequently with other allied health care personnel. Uncertainty and lack of knowledge amongst ophthalmologists about available rehabilitation services were felt to account for the low referral rate of both the more severely visually impaired and their less affected peers for rehabilitative services. Finestone & Gold (1959) discovered in a study carried out in the United States of America, that over three-quarters of the ophthalmologists in their survey fell into what they termed 'low referral groups', where patients with significant eye defects were not referred for other rehabilitation, including counselling services. To date there have been no comparative studies in the United Kingdom other than the present book which explores the role of the ophthalmologist in breaking bad news, the giving of diagnosis and prognosis and the impact of these factors on long term adjustment. What the American studies may display is the need to establish positive and effective links between ophthalmologists and allied care workers. In the later chapters of this book there is exploration of who may usefully break bad news. The ophthalmologist has an important position in relation to patients' perceptions of him/her, but may be supported in this by allied professionals. There is no reason why the task of disclosing diagnosis could not be shared between ophthalmologist, nurse or rehabilitation worker. The patient can feel doubly held and supported.

Patient's response to registration

Registration has been noted by previous investigators (Fitzgerald, 1970) as being a crucial event for patients, involving an increase in stress and anxiety as the disabled individual begins to take in the permanency and implications of loss of sight. Donnelly (1986) noted that for the 50 respondents in her study who had been registered for between one and three years, and for the 31 who were going through the registration process, over half of both groups defined themselves as upset by the process of registration itself. This may indicate, as previously thought, that time is not a reliable indicator of emotional resolution. The percentage of those who were upset three years after registration were the same as those recently registered. Time did not appear to have lessened the incidence of distress.

The three groups identified in Donnelly's study as being most in need of help immediately following registration were:

1) Women aged 65 years and over. (In the present study this was found to relate to both men and women.) (Refer to Chapter 6 for discussion.)

2) Patients who suffered sudden traumatic visual loss.

3) Where residual vision amounted to light perception or less.

Donnelly, though primarily concerned with those registered blind, concurred with Julie Shaw's finding that patients generally lacked information and advice about the process of registration. Indeed, many seemed unaware of its essentially voluntary role, i.e. allowing patients to exercise choice as to whether or not to be registered. Shaw concluded that avoidable anxiety and concerns could have been resolved by earlier contact with specialist social workers. Some patients stated that they would have benefited from seeing someone sooner and that they were past the crisis of losing their sight by the time help eventually arrived. Over one-third of our group claimed they would have welcomed earlier help and intervention. Furthermore, Shaw's survey also identified social workers lack of knowledge of eye conditions, and of the specific process of registration as being another drawback of the system. Such findings support the view that if generic social workers are to work with visually impaired people, additional post qualifying training would be of benefit (refer to Chapter 6).

As will be discussed later in the text, increasing demand on limited resources in finance and personnel both within the National Health Service and welfare sector may have implications for patient care during the process of registration and at other times. This underlines Cullinan's research (1977) that suggests that under one-third of those entitled to be registered are registered because they are unaware of their entitlement to be registered. These findings purport an under-representation of those who might benefit from help and who either decline to be registered or in some way slip through the net of the welfare/health service system. It should be borne in mind that potentially there is an unknown need amongst the visually impaired population as a whole.

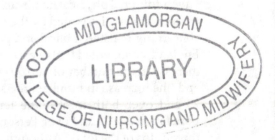

Chapter 3

The Career Begins
Awareness of Sight Loss and Contact with General Practitioner

Introduction

Throughout this book the analogy of a career, generally viewed in society as a positive asset, will be applied to the experience of loss of sight. Clearly, the concept of 'career' for someone who, because of visual impairment, is entering a phase of altered capabilities associated with complex changes and stress is far from a positive experience, particularly when considering that physical handicap may make its presence felt both upon the affected individual and the family. The relevance of this conceptualization for visual impairment has impressed the author sufficiently, with adaption, to utilise this concept of a career in disability.

Julie Shaw has pointed out that the majority of the population may lose a degree of sight as a consequence of ageing, and also that the vast majority have additional physical handicaps or problems apart from loss of sight. The tri-annual statistics issued by the Department of Health and Social Security concerning registered blind and partially sighted persons in March 1986 in England, commented that over the preceding decade there had been a steady increase in the number of persons registered as blind and partially sighted, and 'the increase in numbers registered has been greatest for persons aged 75 and over, both in absolute terms and when expressed as a rate per population age 75 and over. Persons aged 75 and over now account for over three-fifths of the total'. Although minimal loss of sight may be a secondary and potentially less debilitating change for the majority who visit opticians or ophthalmic clinics, and whilst acknowledging that most of us can expect at some time or other in our lives to experience slight problems, the concern in this book is to understand what the experience means for those people who have lost a substantial degree of useful vision and will subsequently be registered either as partially sighted or blind. It is postulated that the career begins when the individual consciously becomes aware of decreasing vision, range, clarity of sight, near or far sighted vision. Arguably, vision can be deteriorating over a far longer period that may be consciously acknowledged. Such awareness of deterioration may threaten internal psychic harmony, cause internal psychic pain or emotional stress, thus suppression of conscious awareness can be viewed as a natural defence mechanism. The time will come when difficulty in seeing can no longer be suppressed or lightly dismissed. It is likely that at this point awareness of changes in vision are consciously registered. Dawning awareness which seemed the common experience for most people in this study was summed up by one lady who lost sight degenerately and was subsequently registered blind:

> 'I noticed it gradually. I used to like to read in the garden but could not indoors, so I went to the optician.'

The sense of hesitation to admit real difficulties was captured in the reflective comment of another lady:

> 'I couldn't see much through my glasses, they seemed dirty to me. I went eventually to the optician and he gave me a letter for my GP.'

Perhaps it was comforting or felt safer to attribute failing sight on dirty spectacles. Such defense mechanisms are a natural human response in the face of anxiety or uncertainty which may be potentially overwhelming. It may also be speculated that the defenses of splitting and projection were unconsciously invoked. The problem was initially projected out onto the glasses; they were seen as the problem.

Defense mechanisms must be viewed and held by giving care with respect and sensitivity. Eventually in most cases reality makes its presence felt. The lady in this example was able to ultimately seek assistance from her general practitioner. Defense mechanisms such as denial can become stuck and counter-productive.

In certain circumstances it appears that individuals may become more attuned or alert to the possibility of visual deterioration where there have been long standing sight difficulties:

> 'I have always had problems with my eyes, and have always had an eye specialist.'

> 'I have been wearing glasses since I was five. I went to my optician regularly. One time he said he couldn't do much for me and gave me a letter for my GP.'

Of the 104 patients in our study, half suspected sight loss prior to diagnosis. It was noted with concern that out of this group 12 had put off or delayed seeking medical advice; all suffered degenerative loss, with eight subsequently registered blind, and four partially sighted. The possible correlation between gradual loss of sight and reluctance to seek medical attention raises speculation. Where sight deteriorates very gradually, often throughout months or years, the day to day effect on the patient's lifestyle and coping ability may be minimal. Avoidance or denial of the change becomes that much easier. The general social idiom that 'left to its own devices the body will sort itself out' or 'the problem will go away', could account in part for the delay in seeking medical attention. However, the majority of visually impaired people lose sight during their middle-to-late years, resulting in a tendency for failing eye sight to be defined as an inescapable part of the inevitable ageing process. There may be, therefore, the social expectation that people should display resignation and stoicism at such times. The consequence of this expectation may be that patients delay seeking help, although suspecting sight loss, because they themselves view this deterioration as the price they must pay for growing old. These under-lying assumptions were sadly echoed in this gentleman's comment about his general practitioner:

'He did not care. All he said was that when people get to 40 years old their eyes start to deteriorate.'

When visual difficulties are brought to full consciousness, the manner in which an individual chooses to respond to the situation will depend largely on pre-existing characteristics of personality, past and present life experien-ces, relationships to important others, upbringing, education and interaction with the wider society.

Sadly, for the 12 who actively put off seeking medical attention, the outcome might have been ameliorated had they sought earlier attention. Although the group is too small to permit firm conclusions, the experiences of this group suggest that there needs to be a shift of public and professional awareness of the implications of early deterioration, however slight. It would be of help in such instances for a health awareness programme to educate the public that loss of sight is not necessarily an inevitable and inescapable part of the ageing process. We all have to take some measure of responsibility for sustaining our physical well being. By encouraging people, despite their fears and hesitation, to seek early medical attention, preventative intervention may be made possible. Such a campaign was launched recently by the British Glaucoma Society.

Within the present study, five patients lost their sight suddenly (traumati-cally). This group had little or no warning of sight loss or time to prepare. Diamond et al (1945) suggest that the severity and suddenness of loss may, in itself, remove false hopes or fantasies about restoration of sight; and in the fullness of time this may facilitate a healthier adjustment to visual impairment. However, contemporary theories on grief reactions to loss uphold the contrary view. Suddenness of loss, it is suggested, with no time to prepare or to begin anticipatory mourning, may lead to a more severe reaction, initially giving rise to greater likelihood of denial and disbelief.

A patient who was referred for counselling following traumatic sight loss through an assault, held ostensively onto the belief for three years prior to the referral that as he had lost his sight so suddenly and, in his perception, so inexplicably, then likewise his sight would return one day, equally as suddenly. Therefore he rejected rehabilitation.

The need for increased inter-professional co- operation and liaison between general practitioners, opticians and ophthalmic clinics became apparent from discussions with some of the patients. Whilst it is reasonable and accepted good practice that general practitioners might want a routine eye test via an optician before making a referral to the hospital, the potential delays at each stage in this process, though well intentioned, may have unforeseen consequences and prolong anxiety for patients. If such a procedure is to be followed, the patient needs to know the reason for such examinations, and as far as possible, what the procedure entails and what may be expected of them. During this pre-diagnostic stage patients may experience heightened anxiety and uncertainty about what the future holds. Collaboration between the professionals involved, linked to sensitive handling of routine pre-diagnostic examinations, may avoid the likelihood of patients feeling unnecessarily vulnerable, as implied by two patients who reminisced:

> 'My eyes were getting worse. I went to my GP, he sent me to the optician, who sent me back to the GP. My GP gave me a letter for the hospital.'

> 'Not satisfied with my optician, I changed him and was told by a second optician that I needed to go to see a specialist. He sent me to my own doctor.'

Although this study did not endeavour to explore or evaluate the role of the optician during this phase, a recurring lament from opticians was that they feel they had too little discussion with either general practitioners or hospital services. One optician, in discussion with the author, cynically reported that in his and other colleagues' experience, too frequently, despite having monitored patients' eye sight throughout months or years, once an optician made a referral to either the general practitioner or ophthalmic clinic, rarely did they receive any feedback from those colleagues about the patients' progress. Further more, it was felt that patients would come back to their optician because they felt more likely to receive an understandable explanation about their eye condition. Whilst this sad perception does not directly relate to this study, it does seem to emphasise Greenblatt's view (1986) that there is too much potentially unhelpful professional insularity amongst those caring for the visually impaired (refer also to Chapter 4).

General Practitioner Services

Encouragingly it was noted that over half the group (59) were satisfied with the way their general practitioner dealt with them. Many spoke appreciatively of the care they had received:

> 'GP was very good and helpful.'

> 'Quite satisfied. He gave me a letter, that is all he can do.'

It was felt by 52 patients that their general practitioner had been sympathetic. Amongst the complimentary comments were:

> 'My doctor said it's a pity you got it so young. My doctor was sympathetic.'

> 'She was one in a million.'

> 'He is very nice. . . gave me a handkerchief.'

Only eight patients were dissatisfied with the service received from their general practitioner, with a further ten feeling they had been dealt with unsympathetically. Three patients lamented:

> 'I got on quite well with my GP. We have argued but he is reasonably good. I felt, however, he could not get rid of me quick enough as he knew there was something seriously wrong with my sight.'

> 'I try not to go and see him very often.'

> 'My doctor gave me no help—said it was my diabetes. I walked out and went to see the hospital doctor who dealt with my diabetes.'

There was a level of concern on the part of patients interviewed lest they pester or waste their general practitioner's time unnecessarily.

It was notable, however, that approximately one-third of the total group, in evaluating satisfaction with their general practitioner, declined to comment either way. Some 31 were unable to say whether or not their general practitioner was sympathetic, whilst 16 could not remember whether or not their general practitioner had been sympathetic. There was no marked variation in this pattern between the respective general practitioner services of the two participating authorities. However, the qualitative answers given by patients frequently contradicted their earlier answers to closed questions on this topic. Off the record, patients were often much more vocal in criticising their general practitioners; although underlying this trend it also appeared they were simultaneously reluctant or guilty to openly criticise their general practitioners. These patients showed preoccupation that they should not be seen as ungrateful, overly-demanding or troublesome. Although this issue was not explored at a greater depth because of time constraints, it was felt that these concerns inhibited and possibly affected patients' overt evaluations. These implicit contradictions are hinted at in the anomalous findings that more patients reported being satisfied with their general practitioner than thought he/she was sympathetic see Table 3.1).

Are we to summarize from this that patients are generally satisfied with the manner in which they are dealt with, even if they do not feel that their general practitioner is sympathetic? The patient who visits his/her general practitioner is taking the first step along a potentially difficult road. The manner in which patients are dealt with at this early stage may be crucial to their overall sense of well-being in a potentially difficult and ultimately alien situation. If at this pre-diagnostic stage the visually impaired individual is dealt with sensitively, enabling him/her to extend or develop a rapport with the general practitioner, then the ground work is done for positive contact later on, once the strain of change and the realisation of loss has been internally registered. Therefore, it seems justified to be concerned about those who go away dissatisfied or unhappy from the contact made with their general practitioner, although it is also recognised that this group is in the minority see Table 3.1).

Table 3.1. Index of Satisfaction with general practitioner

	Positive reply	Negative reply	Don't know/no reply	Total
My GP was sympathetic about my anxiety	51%	13%	36%	100%
My GP understood my feelings about my difficulty in seeing	45%	14%	41%	100%
Was he sympathetic/unsympathetic	50%	5%	45%	100%
Did he seem interested/disinterested	52%	9%	39%	100%
Satisfied with the way GP dealt with me at that time	56%	9%	35%	100%

Over one-third of the patients gave positive responses to all five questions. A further quarter had more positive than negative responses. One-tenth of patients gave more negative than positive responses. This group were more dissatisfied with their general practitioner than the rest of the patients interviewed.

In general, there were no significant differences between the patients who were satisfied with their general practitioners and those who were not. Men tended to be more satisfied than women; those over 80 years old were the least satisfied age group. The partially sighted were more dissatisfied than the blind. Those whose sight problem was traumatic in origin were more satisfied than those whose sight loss was degenerative, which may suggest that in crisis appropriate intervention with regards to sympathy and medical cover were more likely to have been available. Perhaps when sight diminishes gradually, usually in later years, the need for particular sympathy and space for discussion is more likely to be overlooked, particularly as a consequence of hard pressed general practitioners and ever growing case loads. Overall the implication is that women of 80 years old and over with degenerative partial sight were the most dissatisfied group.

Chapter 4

The Career Progresses
Contact with the Ophthalmologist

Introduction

This chapter explores the role of the ophthalmologist in determining the psychological management of patients who are losing their sight. By considering the results from this study and patients' perception of care given, as opposed to clinical treatment received (with which this book does not concern itself), the aim is to consider the constraints and boundaries within which the doctor/patient relationship operates.

The chapter will conclude with a brief diagnostic discussion about what may constitute a positive, enabling interaction between doctor and patient. Recommendations for the psychological management of visually impaired patients will be offered.

Seeing the ophthalmologist and having the condition explained

The ophthalmologist can be instrumental in influencing patients' response both during the onset of loss of sight and later during registration and rehabilitation. The ability of patients to take in the actuality and possible finality of loss of sight will, broadly speaking, be in direct relationship to the manner in which the patient is prepared for and told the bad news. In the case of sudden (traumatic) loss there might be little time to prepare, though the intensity of violence of the loss may, in itself, reinforce the irreversibility of the eye condition. Patients who lose sight traumatically, however, are a small minority within the visually impaired population. Only 7 percent of the total in this study had lost sight traumatically. In some ways then, this group might pose fewer ethical and personal dilemmas for the ophthalmologist than degenerative patients when debating when, what and how much to tell patients. These are crucial factors determining the quality of patients' overall adjustment.

In order to gain a clearer understanding of how patients felt they had been dealt with by ophthalmology services, and to chart their progress through the hospital system, we asked how long they had to wait between the initial consultation with the ophthalmologist and having their eye condition (diagnosis) explained. The results from this question were difficult to interpret because some patients may have had two or three consultations prior to diagnosis being made, and because frequently there are considerable gaps between out patient appointments. However, 11 patients waited six months or more for an explanation and, more worrying, three stated that they had waited over a year. Unnecessary delays in talking to patients about their eye condition is reprehensible. In the previous chapter we considered patients' heightened anxiety when seeking medical assistance. Fluctuating levels of anxiety and stress may affect patients as they progress in their career. Delays in explanation of diagnosis do nothing to alleviate this understandable response.

Of greatest concern was the fact that 12 patients asserted that they had never received an explanation about their eye condition. One blind female patient stated:

> 'The hospital said they could not do any more, so I would have to live with it, but I would have liked to know why this was happening to me'.

Another partially sighted female said:

> 'I can't remember his ever explaining it (diagnosis) to me.'

An explanation of this non-occurrence could be that patients may choose to be selectively non-hearing when being told about their diagnosis. However, whilst this possibility undermines the patient's plausibility as a witness of his/her own experience, by giving such perceptions the benefit of the doubt, it follows that there needs to be discussion about why patients may not be told the truth or facts about their condition, or at least why there is hesitation about talking more openly with patients:

> 'I was left completely in the dark, (notice the apt analogy) I had to ask for an explanation'.
>
> (Male, blind, 65-79)

A familiar response from some ophthalmologists is that they do not want to destroy hope; that the patient will not be able to cope with the disclosure. Or, who knows what medical technological advances may prove possible in the future. It is suggested that such a response may indicate an emotional defence towards dealing with the unpleasant task of breaking bad news; therefore, the human response and tendency is to avoid or distort the facts. This might be an unconscious process, or rationalized consciously as protecting the patient. Certainly, the patient's emotional defences need to be respected and insight gently disclosed to the patient. As will be seen later in the case presentations of Mary and Lottie (Chapter 7), to leave false hopes does the patient a disservice. An individual cannot begin to adjust unless they know what it is they must potentially face and adjust to. False hope may set up unrealistic expectations and undermine motivation to participate in rehabilitation.

On a more positive note, just under half the group (50 patients) were given their diagnosis within one month following the initial consultation. It should also be remembered that disclosure of diagnosis may be delayed pending the results of medical investigations.

Was adequate information given about diagnosis

The complexity and difficulty of considering concepts such as adequacy/inadequacy, which are inherently value-laden and necessarily subjective constructs, should be borne in mind. The interpretation of these concepts may change from one individual to another. For example, a doctor may sincerely feel that he has given an adequate explanation of diagnosis in keeping with his philosophy and standards. The patient, on the other hand, may feel baffled by medical jargon and consequently perceive the explanation as inadequate. The patient, who is on the receiving end of the exchange, may be grossly affected by the content of the message, which has life changing implications. The patient's perceptions should therefore be given attention. Every effort should be made to provide an explanation that the patient can grasp and personally judges to be adequate.

Encouragingly, 46 patients felt they were given adequate information. Just under one-third of the group (30 patients), however, felt they had received an inadequate explanation about their diagnosis from their specialist. The remainder of the group (28 patients) were unable to comment either way. Comments ranged from:

Adequate

> 'Left eye completely gone. The retina has gone. We do not know why, nothing can be done. It has shut up like a venetian blind. Right eye, like a mirror when the backing has come off, that is what is happening, it will get worse.'
>
> (Female, blind, 65–79).

> 'I told him that my sister had tear duct trouble, and he said "yes, that is what is wrong with your eyes too".'
>
> (Female, partially sighted, degenerative).

> 'The hospital doctor said my eye was so severely damaged it was irreparable—my other eye was still good at this time.'
>
> (Female, blind, degenerative).

Inadequate

> 'Didn't explain, said he would register instantly, no further information given.'
>
> (Male, partially sighted, degenerative).

'The doctor said that I had neglected my eye.'

(Female, partially sighted, degenerative).

'He just said it was cataract. I heard from other people what cataract is.'

(Male, blind, degenerative).

'Just told me it was glaucoma.'

(Male, blind, degenerative).

Giving information in response to patients' needs or questions is an acknowledgement of the patients' right to have feelings concerning that information, and to make of it what they will, either to assimilate the information, working through it, or to selectively block out the message. Once the information (diagnosis) and explanation of it are sensitively supplied, then the patient may exercise choice and may be more able to make informed decisions in consequence.

Some patients were able to explore their responsibility in promoting discussion about their eye condition:

'I blame myself; I should have asked more questions.'

(Male, partially sighted, degenerative, 65–79).

'If you ask questions, you get answers.'

(Female, blind, degenerative, 40–64).

It is debatable whether the onus of responsibility should be on the patients to encourage their doctors to share information. The relationship between doctor and patient is generally agreed to be an unequal one, insomuch as many patients potentially feel too shy and diffident to question the doctor. It takes a certain type of person, some would say determined, who at a time of potential stress can push for details when information may be unforthcoming. Some patients appeared confused about the distinction between the adequacy of explanation and the sort of medical treatment received. For example:

'I was given immaculate treatment, exemplary, but it was never really fully explained to me, I was told it was a blood clot.'

(Female, blind, trauma, 65–79).

Over half the group (60 patients) felt that the explanation of diagnosis was understandable. This would seem to suggest that when information is given it is likely to be comprehensible, though not perhaps always adequate. It is notable that 24 patients (23%) were unable to comment on the comprehensibility of diagnosis. It appeared that for those losing their sight gradually, understanding the explanation of diagnosis seemed a greater problem; of the 14 patients who did not feel the diagnosis was understandable, 12 had suffered degenerative (gradual) loss of sight.

Just under half the group felt they had received consistent information about their loss of sight from the different doctors who saw them. It was nevertheless a matter of concern that 21 patients (one in five) felt they had received conflicting information about their diagnosis and prognosis from the different doctors seen. This may be explained in part by the team approach adopted in most out patient clinics. In such instances patients may only see the consultant ophthalmologist at the initial consultation, but thereafter the patient may progress down the hierarchy, seeing registrars, house officers, or whoever is available from the team to attend particular clinics. In such circumstances it is conceivable that a junior doctor may not have the experience or professional authority to disclose detailed information, and so may hesitate to respond to patients' questions. Consequently, inconsistent explanations and sometimes contradictory or conflicting information may be given to patients. Early, well intentioned reassurance given by staff may be overturned by a fuller account given later by the ophthalmologist, which also may contribute to inconsistent information. Julie Shaw reported that 4 percent of the 104 in her group criticised that there was 'no continuity of doctors seen'. One means of averting the possibility of inconsistent information being given, which must surely leave patients and families confused and uncertain about what their eye condition entails, might be the establishment of a key worker system of care within the clinic structure and the management of patients. In this way the patient would have a greater likelihood of seeing the same doctor at each appointment.

The ophthalmologist would always retain overall responsibility for the patient, but could advise and oversee the key doctor/patient relationship. This tightening up of patient management might have several benefits for both patient and doctor. By ensuring that the patient meets the same doctor at every appointment, the environment and opportunity for greater rapport is provided. In these circumstances the doctor may get to know the patient in a more personal manner, and thus be more likely to be able to respond helpfully and in a positive way to the patients needs for medical (clinical) assistance and emotional support. In other words, a holistic approach of treating the whole person rather than merely clinical signs and symptoms, becomes more possible. Assistance which addresses the emotional as well

Table 4.1. Did the ophthalmologist help prepare patients for sight loss?

	<64		65-67		80+		Not Stated		Total	
	No.	%	No.	%	No.	%	No.	%	No.	%
Yes	4	22	6	18	7	18	1	7	18	17
No	9	50	21	64	20	51	8	58	58	56
Don't know	2	11	0	-	5	13	2	14	9	9
No answer	3	17	6	18	7	18	3	21	19	18
Total group	18	100	33	100	39	100	14	100	104	100

as the physical is more likely to be perceived by the patient as effective (see Table 4.1).

Over half the group (58 patients) felt that their ophthalmologist had not helped them to prepare for loss of sight. Clearly, there are heavy demands on doctors' time in a busy out-patient clinic. However, the manner in which patients are helped to prepare for sight loss is bound up with the way diagnosis and prognosis are explained. Without a sensitive, but realistic, explanation of their condition, patients cannot begin to grasp the changes they may be faced with. Open discussion with both patients and families about the diagnosis is therefore an integral part of preparation for sight loss. Of the above group, most were 65 years old or older. Though these results are consistent with the age distribution within the study, only 18 were aged under 65 in all. Whether patients in their middle to late years receive less preparation as a result of the philosophy that loss of sight is part of the ageing process should be considered. Donnelly's (1986) study also highlights the need for increased support for the over 65s. It could be argued that the elderly might require and benefit from even greater preparation and rehabilitation, because they have become more set in their ways and established lifestyle patterns. Any major trauma or life event may cause greater disruption because the older person is less adaptable than a younger person whose life stretches before them, and who has not, perhaps, become too set in their ways.

Following the anticipated mourning process, the younger patient may feel a greater spur to actively participate in rehabilitation programs because there is a prevailing sense that life has to be lived. The younger disabled person may have a family to support and unfulfilled ambitions, all of which may add to motivation. Frequently, on the other hand, there may be a prevailing attitude amongst some elderly people that there is no point in rehabilitation as they have lived their life. Rehabilitation, though able to increase independence and bring possible benefits such as increased confidence and self esteem, may be viewed as understandably irksome and stressful, particularly for those over the age of 70.

Within both participating authorities over half the group (56%) reported that their doctors had not helped them prepare; this suggests a similarity in the way doctors respond to this dilemma. Forty-eight patients (46%) felt that their specialist did not take time to discuss any difficulties with them. Patients related instances of diagnosis being given with no back up support being made available to talk through the situation:

'I was very depressed. I needed someone to take the time and trouble to sit down and explain it all to me. The hospital just left me. . . they told me, and then they told me to go home, I was just left. If someone had sat and talked to me and explained it, it would have helped. . . would have helped tremendously.'

(Male, blind, degenerative, 40–64)

Other replies, though less dramatic, indicated general dissatisfaction concerning both discussion of difficulties and preparation for loss of sight:

'to have more time given by the doctors.' (Female, partially sighted, degenerative, 80+).

Many spoke repeatedly of being unable to prepare. In this group, replies also suggested a sense of shock or unexpectedness for what was to come:

'I was not able to prepare. It came as a great shock.'

(Female, blind, degenerative).

'No, I never expected to lose my good eye.'

(Female, partially sighted, degenerative).

A picture emerges which suggests that, on the one hand, patients may be told little or nothing about their diagnosis, or be told openly about their condition with apparently insufficient or no time to talk through their response and questions. One lady summed up these types of explanation by saying:

'No, the doctor (ophthalmologist) was too blunt, but I saw another lady doctor and she explained it all to me and was very good'.

(Female, partially sighted, degenerative).

Some comfort can be drawn from the 18 patients who felt their ophthalmologist had helped them prepare; their comments were justly appreciative of the assistance offered:

'I saw about six different specialists, and had long discussions with all of them.'

(Male, blind, degenerative, 65–79).

'He was marvellous.'

(Male, blind, degenerative).

However, other comments, also from this group, suggested a sense of confusion between emotional assistance in preparing for visual deterioration and preventative treatment or technical assistance offered, as with the supply of visual aids. This type of comment went something like:

'He was really good, suggested glasses but never really explained why my sight was going!'

It may be surmised from such comments that patients feel that their medical and ancillary care is not suffering, which is surely a prime concern. However, if busy and over-pressurized clinics are not allowing the opportunity for doctors and patients to ventilate concerns, it is hardly surprising that over half the group felt unprepared for what was to follow. (Refer to Chapter 5). It was noted that seven patients sought a second opinion, of which five were blind and two partially sighted. It was noted that four specifically sought a second opinion because they felt they had been given inadequate information. It was considered significant that all seven who had sought a second opinion had suffered degenerative loss. (78% of the group suffered degenerative loss). Though not significant in relationship to the total group, the findings from this group may suggest that it is even more crucial for clear, unequivocal information to be given to patients who are losing their sight gradually; especially if they are to be spared unnecessary and fruitless searching for a cure (see Table 4.2). The comment of one lady implies that what she was really searching for was reassurance about future assistance:

> 'The first specialist I saw explained my eye condition, and said nothing more could be done. I did not want to accept this and went to a second specialist who was very nice, explained about aids, etc.'
>
> (Female, blind, degenerative).

Table 4.2. Index of satisfaction with ophthalmologist services

	Positive reply	Negative reply	Don't know/no reply	Total
How did your ophthalmologist explain your eye condition? Was the explanation understandable?	60 (58%)	14 (13%)	30 (29%)	104 (100%)
Do you feel that you were given adequate/inadequate information?	46 (44%)	30 (29%)	28 (27%)	104 (100%)
Did your ophthalmologist help you prepare for your loss of sight?	18 (17%)	58 (56%)	28 (27%)	104 (100%)
Do you feel your ophthalmologist had time to discuss any difficulties with you?	42 (40%)	48 (46%)	14 (13%)	104 (100%)
Were you given the same information by the different doctors that you saw?	46 (44%)	21 (20%)	37 (36%)	104 (100%)
Overall, could this experience have been improved for you?	50 (48%) 'no–experience could not have been improved.'	25 (24%0 'yes–experience could have been improved.'	29 (28%)	104 (100%)

Could the hospital experience have been improved?

Although just under half the interviewed group (50 patients) considered that the hospital experience could not have been improved, just under one quarter (25 patients) felt the experience could have been better. Their criticism appeared to relate to both practical and emotional help required at that time:

'Someone giving practical information. I would also have appreciated counselling.'

(Male, partially sighted, trauma).

'Better and quicker diagnosis. I had tests for all sorts of things before they realized the problem was with my eyes.'

(Male, blind, degenerative')

'By talking to someone or having someone to talk to about it.'

(Female, partially sighted, degenerative).

It was difficult to establish whether this dissatisfaction relates to patients' psychological and emotional experiences of this phase, because loss of sight is so personally distressing, or whether the services in reality did little to diminish their distress.

The intervention at this juncture, if not earlier, of a medical social worker or specialist worker for the visually impaired, with requisite counselling skills, could do much to alleviate anxiety, answer questions, and liaise with medical and community services. The social worker would potentially have a different relationship with the client than the doctor/patient relationship permits. The social worker/client interaction may not be encumbered by guilt that they are unable to restore eye sight, which is a possible factor in the doctor/patient interchange. Referral to an experienced social worker for psycho-social assessment should be an integral part of the diagnostic clinic's routine management of patients.

Such a procedure could potentially forestall the sad reflections of one lady summing up her hospital experiences eighteen months post-registration:

'If I had someone to talk to about my loss of sight; I would have appreciated psychological help, to discuss emotional problems, e.g. anger and grief. Right now I feel I would still like and appreciate this help.'

(Female, blind, degenerative).

The Doctor/Patient relationship and potential for change

Earlier in this chapter the important and central role that the ophthalmologist may assume to assist the patient's understanding and implications of failing eyesight was considered. The uniqueness of this relationship, about which much has been documented elsewhere, encourages the patient, who is in the passive dependent position, to place trust and confidence in the consultant. The doctor may unconsciously represent a primary figure from childhood, for instance the father of the patient. Such subtle potential components of the relationship provide the environment and opportunity for the ophthalmologist to positively influence patients' perceptions and response to loss of sight. The sensitive psychological management of the patient may entail the ophthalmologist allowing additional time in clinic to talk through the treatment plan with the patient, outlining the reasons for specific investigations. If, prior to formal diagnosis, there is a significant concern about poor long term visual prognosis, the consultant might begin to gently prepare the patient for change by sounding out what the patient thinks, or fears, is happening to his/her sight, exploring to what degree the condition is affecting the patient at home, at work, with social routine, etc. In this manner, whilst not assailing the patient's psychological defence or destroying all hope, the ophthalmologist is sensitively sowing a seed of doubt, gently preparing the patient for possible change. As stated earlier, in conjunction with this preliminary phase it would be beneficial for the patient to be assured of access to a specialist medical or community social worker.

Later, when giving the diagnosis, the consultant needs to give the patient a clear explanation in non-technical language, perhaps using visual aids or simple diagrams, to clarify the damage and to assist retention of the facts in the patient's mind. At every stage in the relationship the patient should be encouraged to ask questions and seek information, with reassurance that additional appointments can be made for further discussion. A follow up appointment a week or two after disclosure of diagnosis or prognosis allows the patient time to digest information and to recover from the immediate shock which may well be present. In this way there is a greater likelihood that the patient will feel sustained and individually respected.

The patient brings to the doctor/patient relationship expectations, or at least hope of a cure or healing, which must affect the doctor's response when he is no longer able to offer effective medical intervention. Because of these preoccupations within the relationship, perhaps the doctor is not the best person to break the bad news. However, he could rather use his influence with the patient by acting as a confirmer of information given.

Counselling and inter-personal communication skills is given minimal place in the training curriculum of most medical schools. The emphasis, and some would say quite rightly, is placed on technical skill for clinical practice. If, however, the medical fraternity in general, and ophthalmologists in particular, insist on retaining the total responsibility for breaking bad news, then a shift of emphasis in selection and training, encompassing communication and counselling skills, would be desirable.

It would also be beneficial to both patients and doctors if attention were given to staffing levels, and patient/staff ratios, particularly with reference to the centralisation of specialist intervention within an area health authority and in pressurized urban clinics.

Recommendations

1. The instigation of a key worker approach in clinics would increase the likelihood of consistent information being given to patients and facilitate rapport and good communication.

2. There is a need for more time to be allocated to doctors to talk through the implications of diagnosis and prognosis, in order to help prepare the patient, both emotionally and practically, for the onset of visual impairment.

3. Patient referral to an experienced social worker for psycho-social assessment, counselling or information giving, should be an integral part of the diagnostic clinic's routine management of patients, thus allowing the appropriate liaison between medical and statutory services.

4. Additional follow up appointments need to be available for recapitulation of disclosure, one or two weeks after initial diagnosis or prognosis has been given.

5. The ophthalmologist is not necessarily the best or only person to break bad news. Benefit for both patient and doctor may be gained from the ophthalmologist sharing responsibility either within the team or with an experienced social worker.

6. There needs to be a shift of emphasis in the selection and training of doctors and ophthalmologists—the training curriculum of medical schools would benefit from greater awareness of counselling and communication skills.

7. Patient/staff ratios need to be re-evaluated in the light of current centralisation policies within health provision planning, if unnecessary distress is to be averted for patients.

Chapter 5

Registration

'A Point of No Return?'

Introduction

Partial or total loss of sight is a 'condition' uniquely experienced by each individual, family and friends. The effects of visual impairment will have potential repercussions on every facet of living: social status, identity, employment, finance, relationships and behaviour. Vision can deteriorate rapidly within days or weeks, (traumatic loss) or throughout months or years[1] (degenerative loss). The origins of deterioration may be rooted in specific ophthalmic conditions such as macular degeneration, glaucoma or cataracts; or, quite commonly, constitute part of a systemic physical ailment as in multiple-sclerosis or diabetes. In the latter instance the individual is having to respond to a complexity of changes and loss of physical function. In such cases loss of vision and registration itself may assume only a small part of other more disturbing changes to be faced, and as such may assume, by comparison, less importance. Therefore, wherever possible in the study, special note was made of additional disabilities which might have a bearing on patients' replies.[2]

Registration of the blind evolved out of the 1920 Blind Person's Act. The partially sighted were later included in this process following the 1948 National Assistance Act. Essentially, local authority social services departments were deemed responsible for compiling and maintaining a record of all visually impaired inhabitants within their local area. Registration was instigated to identify and promote the welfare of these two groups. In this way visual handicap has been singled out for social labelling, when compared to other forms of physical incapacitation for which there is no similar procedure. The established 'green card status' noting physical incapacitation for employment purposes is voluntary and commonly held to be somewhat arbitrary in definition. Administered by the Department of Social Security, this categorization does not give or ensure automatic access to assistance

---

[1] For the purpose of this study, traumatic loss relates to the period from onset, within days or weeks, up to six months. Degenerative loss relates to onset from six months up to several years.

[2] 29 patients (28%) had some level of hearing impairment. Nine percent had other disabilities.

from social services, nor are additional specialist benefits guaranteed in consequence.

The process of registration under the 1940 Employment Act as physically handicapped is voluntary, dependent on a general practitioner's or specialist's collaborating report. In practice it is common for applicants to attend an independent examination arranged by the Department of Health and Social Security. As will be explored later in the text, registration as visually impaired, although officially voluntary, can happen without patients seemingly being aware of it.

The statutory definition of blind registration is that a person must be 'so blind as to be unable to perform any work for which eyesight is essential' (National Assistance Act 1948).

The blind categorization, broadly speaking, considers the visual acuity range of 3/60 or less to denote suitability for registration.

The advised definition of partial sight given by the Ministry of Health is one who is:

> not blind within the meaning of the Act of 1948 but who is nevertheless substantially and permanently handicapped by congenitally defective vision in whose case illness or injury has caused defective vision of a substantial and permanently handicapping character. (Circular 4/55 Ministry of Health Appendices III and IV) [3]

Here the visual acuity range of 6/60 meters applies. Assessment for both partial sight or blindness is also generally dependent on field of vision and/or prognosis.

Eligibility for registration can only be determined by a consultant ophthalmologist. If appropriate, form BD8, which sets the process of registration in motion, is completed and forwarded to the Director of Social Services for inclusion on the register and for statistical purposes. It is at this stage, theoretically, that local specialist or generic social workers are informed about the registration, so that an assessment can be arranged. The Chronically Sick and Disabled Persons Act 1970 enjoins local authorities to ensure that visually impaired people understand the range of local services and benefits available to which they may be entitled following registration as blind or partially sighted. However, as Shaw (1985) comments from her survey of local authorities service provision to the visually handicapped: 'in two of the nineteen local authorities participatint. . . it was evident that a significant proportion of clients referred. . . via form BD8 would not necessarily receive a visit'. As Shaw suggests from her survey, it is necessary to bear in mind that not all the visually handicapped will have access to specialist assessment or rehabilitation. Furthermore, as discussed in the two preceding chapters, the time spent in assessing and talking to clients about diagnosis and preparing them for taking in the news of registration is very

---

[3] No Statutory definition could be traced.

important, as is the time factor involved in visiting a client at home following registration. If there is, for example, a three month delay between receipt of BD8 forms within the social services departments and an assessment interview being arranged, then the client has not only had to cope in the interim in the best way he or she can, but may also have improvised coping techniques, both practically and emotionally, which are potentially counterproductive and, because entrenched, become more difficult to alter. This might apply to the client who, for example, has become inappropriately dependent on family. The circularity of this well- intentioned collusion (bolstered up by lack of knowledge/experience about the potential capabilities of visually impaired people) serves to reinforce the client's view of himself as helpless and dependent. We will be exploring such experiences later in this chapter (refer also to Chapter 8.)

Another general issue concerning registration is that there is no standardised procedure laid down for inclusion. Despite the guidelines contained on form BD8 as previously quoted, there is such scope for the ophthalmologist's individual interpretation about if or when to register patients. Cullinan (1977) points to the consequence of 'under' registration. Many factors may account for either non-registration or delayed registration where it may seem to be appropriate by the affected individual or specialist workers. In the closing sections of this chapter an attempt will be made to hypothesize and explore the possible likelihood and causes of delayed or non- registration. However, such investigation is not easily accessible.

As both Donnelly (1986) and Penelope Shaw highlight in their respective studies, registration is a voluntary procedure which seems little emphasized to potential registrants. One of the aims of this study was to continue evaluation of the doctor/patient relationship, as described by patients who are consumers, exploring how the process and purpose of registration were explained to them, i.e. How were they prepared for registration? What did eligibility for inclusion on the Visually Impaired Register mean to them?

Fitzgerald (in press) has suggested that registration constitutes potentially a point of no return, where the permanency and reality of loss is borne in on the patient. If we concur with this theory that the acceptance of the reality and permanency of loss of sight is crucial to long term adjustment, then it follows that the way news of registration is given and worked through, often following discussion of diagnosis, will be crucial and formative for patients' overall response.

It seemed important to test out an elusive and complex postulate which evolved from the experiences of workers and past clients, but which also appeared to be something of a disquieting myth concerning registration generally; namely, that some patients were not being given a clear explanation of the purpose and implications of registration. Furthermore, it appeared possible that some clients were unaware that they had been registered at all, only finding out when the first contact was made from social services departments. Such complex issues are not easily accessible for consideration. The patient/doctor relationship is clearly underpinned by many factors at any time, but more especially at the point of registration, with such factors as:

- the patient's ability to assimilate or take in the news and attached information;
- the many pressures on ophthalmology clinics, in terms of time allocated to individual patients, staffing ratios, etc.;
- the individual ophthalmologists' experience of and knowledge about registration linked to the corresponding services, benefits and rehabilitation available following registration.

The ophthalmologists' understanding of the potential of visually impaired people is crucial. To what extent the specialist has been in a position to appreciate the capabilities and skills that a visually impaired person can utilize to live as full a life as possible is of paramount importance. Some years ago, for example, a 20 year-old recalled that his failing eyesight was indicated to him by his ophthalmologist, suggesting he give up his chosen professional of banking and take up basket making. On inquiring about this remark he learnt of his poor prognosis and eligibility to be registered as blind. This was an appalling way for such news to be given. This bemused and stunned young man initially feared that such was the occupation open to him because his specialist knew of no other, save this historical stereotype.

The patient's perception and expectation of the ophthalmologist should be explored, whilst weighing up how realistic such expectations may or may not be.

Despite the somewhat daunting nature of the task, it appears appropriate in explaining this subtle relationship to retain such questions when listening to what our patients have to report about this phase of their career.

Several interdependent but distinct factors which are thought likely to help or hinder patients through the process of registration will be explored, relying heavily on patients' moving accounts of this period. The reader is urged to pay special heed to these reflections.

The interval between disclosure of diagnosis and discussion about registration is felt to be central in facilitating preparation for the possibility of registration. Therefore the first half of the investigation will focus on these factors. Patients' reflections about what registration meant to them, its perceived advantages and disadvantages, will also be considered.

The second line of enquiry will consider not only an overview of the time taken to complete all three stages of registration (discussed later in this chapter), but will extend to review clients' perceptions about the range of services received from social service departments, the adequacy and appropriateness of rehabilitation to meet their individual needs.

It is assumed that the process of registration and the rehabilitation service appended thereto, will vary in type and colour from area to area. This chapter seeks to identify common themes and characteristics which will be relevant to our understanding of registration and its effect on individuals, both as patients and clients of the system which seeks to provide a caring service.

Discussion concerning registration

Given the prescribed procedure for registration, one might expect the consultant ophthalmologist to discuss the reasons for and implications of registration with the patient. The results of this study disquietingly suggest a very different trend.

Just under half the patients interviewed (45%) discussed registration with the ophthalmologist. Thirty-one patients (30%) claimed they did not discuss registration with either hospital doctor or nurse. The patients in this group first discussed registration with the identified 'other' specialist worker (outside the hospital system). This suggests that over a third of those patients did not have the opportunity to exercise choice about whether or not they agreed with or wanted to be registered.

In Authority 'B' 22 patients reported that they had first discussed registration with an identified 'other', as against seven patients in Authority 'A'. This suggests that patients in Authority 'B' were less likely to discuss registration with a doctor.

In practice this might usually mean that patients first become aware of registration through contact with their local social services department, with a specialist social worker or technical officer calling to complete the process and to assess the client's needs. It is disturbing to speculate that one-third of the group would have had no prior warning or explanation about the need to become registered as visually impaired. This sizable group appears to have fallen through the hospital net, recalling no opportunity to consider the pros and cons of registration with their consultant. A further point of speculation concerns the remaining 24 patients who could not recall who first discussed registration with them, and the implications of this.

Just under half of the group, 46 patients, were not able to say how long it was after diagnosis that registration was discussed. Of the 58 who were able to remember, 17 were seen within a month, and nearly half within six months. However, nine people had to wait a year before registration was discussed and 11 people stated that it was never discussed at all, although they were all registered:

> 'I did not know I had been registered. I only know that the lady had written a letter to X. I can't remember who first told me I'd been registered. I can't remember ever discussing registration with anyone.'

> 'I did not know it had happened.'

> 'I was not told specifically that I was to be registered.'

It is possible that patients might have been told something about registration but chose to be selectively non-hearing, to deny or block out such information. However, it should be of fundamental concern that it is the patient's perceptions which are central to this investigation. Therefore, we must assume that some patients are not being given an explanation and are thus denied the opportunity to use registration in a constructive manner; asking necessary questions of their consultant, taking in the answers and working through such insight.

It will be seen from Table 5.1 that, perhaps not surprisingly, registration tended to be discussed sooner with blind people than with the partially sighted. Of the 58 patients who could remember, discussion took place within a month for 11 people registered blind, compared with six partially sighted. Over half the blind group (17 patients) had discussed registration within six months compared with just over a third of the partially sighted group (nine patients).

Table 5.1. Time of discussion of registration by extent of sight loss

Length of time	Blind		Partially sighted		Total	
	No.	%	No.	%	No.	%
Within one month	11	35	6	23	17	29
Within six months	6	19	4	12	10	17
Within one year	6	19	5	19	11	19
Over one year	5	16	4	15	9	16
Never discussed	3	10	8	31	11	19
TOTAL	31	100	27	100	58	100
Don't know, can't remember	17		11		28	
No answer	10		8		18	
TOTAL GROUP	56		47		104	100

Among the 11 who had never discussed registration with their consultant, it is interesting to note that eight of these were partially sighted. This might suggest that partial loss of sight is presumed by ophthalmologists to be less socially and emotionally disrupting, and therefore less pressing or necessary for discussion. For this group who were not told of registration, consultants might be avoiding the difficult and time consuming process of breaking news such as this. As mentioned in the preceding chapter, the involvement of the specialist/medical social worker to assist the ophthalmologist and to share the task of imparting news of eligibility for registration might forestall such omissions and oversights. At this point the social worker would be able to make an early assessment of need, provide basic information about services and, more important, refer the client to the area team for on- going support and rehabilitation, in this way circumventing possible delays in the administrative process of registration.

Just under two-thirds of the group (68 patients) evaluated the adequacy of discussion concerning registration. The remaining 36 patients felt unable to comment either way. Of the 42 patients who found the discussion adequate, a larger proportion were blind (27 patients), as opposed to 15 partially sighted. Perhaps the greater the sight loss the easier it is to accept registration.

Just under a quarter of those interviewed, 25 patients, reported that discussion of registration had been inadequate. Patients' assessment of inadequacy did not appear to be related to the extent of sight loss, as the dissatisfied patients in this group were evenly divided between blind and partially sighted.

A higher proportion of the 80+ age group were not able to comment on the adequacy of discussion concerning registration, which might in some ways be indicative of elderly patients having to recall experience from previous months. However, it could also imply that more elderly clients required additional assistance and time to assimilate dialogue and to accept encouragement to take up and use services. Because numbers are so small in the individual age bands within the study, it is difficult to draw firm conclusions. However, the under 65s appeared to be less satisfied with the adequacy of explanation than those aged 65 and over.

The younger patients might have different and more exacting expectations of their ophthalmologist. The sense of greater dissatisfaction amongst the under 65's might also reflect their realistic concern for a greater level of information to assist them in making adaptive plans, especially pertinent for those still in employment who have not yet retired. However, such matters have to remain speculative, but might underlie the need for further discussion within this group also. The following two quotations were fairly typical of the 80+ age group who were uncertain what registration meant:

'I didn't realize what it (registration) meant. I thought it meant being given a white stick.'

'I was so dazed at the time, I just could not take it in, so could not really say what I thought about the explanation the doctor gave.'

Patient's feelings about registration as visually impaired

The range, type and intensity of feelings that each patient may experience following loss of sight will depend on a constellation of factors. Such influences might include their previous knowledge, experience, value judgments and attitudes towards the disabled in general and the visually impaired in particular. The response and attitudes of family and friends to the patient's altered capabilities may intensify and influence the emotional and psychological response of the disabled person. These external or social dynamics are simultaneously and continuously interacting with the patient's internal psychological world. The system of the patient's internal world comprises the sum total of previous life experiences, losses, changes, relationship to others, self identity, aspirations and behaviour, culminating in the view of self; why a person is as he/she is at any given time in response to particular circumstances. The meeting of the external social world with the internal emotional and psychological system will ultimately determine how the individual reacts to the changes which visual deterioration imposes.

Furthermore, loss of sight, whether partial or total, constitutes a significant sensory deprivation. Ninety percent of the information we collect and process about the world around us and our relationship to it is conveyed through our eyes and sight. A major part of our interaction and relationships to other human beings is transmitted and received through non-verbal communication with eye contact being a central component of non-verbal dialogue. The visually impaired person may become insidiously socially isolated because the nuances of such communication are lost (Hicks (1981), Hall (1982)), or because loss of sight results in mobility difficulties. The affected individual may experience problems getting around independently unassisted and in consequence become housebound and cut off from society. (These themes will be elaborated further in Chapter 6 concerning psychosocial adjustment.)

All the aforementioned factors may ultimately impinge on and influence how the patient feels about being registered as visually impaired, with the attendant implication that loss of sight is 'here to stay'. Up to the time of registration it is conceivable that many patients may live with false hope, anticipating that the doctor will 'do' or administer something to cure or take the sight problem away. Such a possibility is supported and given credence by the 58 patients in this study, over half the group, who felt their ophthalmologist had not helped them prepare for the loss of sight:

> 'Could not take it in, kept hoping if they gave me drops it would be alright.'

> 'I felt it was all a mistake and they could do more for me, they were very blunt when they said no more could be done.'

The evaluation of the patient's emotional response to registration is central to the aim of this study, i.e. to investigate patient/clients' wider psychological, emotional and social response to loss of sight. The poignant and revealing comments of patients in this study can teach us much about the far reaching consequences of and psychological response to visual impairment, and the process of registration which to date has been under-investigated.

As might be expected, patients' experiences and sentiments about registration differed widely in content and degree. The replies broadly fell into four categories which encapsulated the continuum of feelings about registration:

1. Acute Psycho-Social Distress

This was the most prevalent within the study, forming the commonest reoccurring theme of all patients' replies. Most of the patients interviewed expressed feelings of shock, numbness and disbelief about becoming registered:

> 'Shocked when told I was to be registered as a blind person. I was not conscious of being that bad.'

> 'Shock. I felt it was just procedure for them and what would follow. The consultant said he was unsure what was available in this area.'

> 'Shocked initially, but realised later that this was likely to have happened.' 'Registration—came as a great shock.'

As might be anticipated, tearfulness, agitation and anxiety were frequently present, particularly in the early days or weeks following registration when feelings of despair, inadequacy and frustration also abounded:

> 'The doctor told me, I would never be able to see again, I cried all the time.'
>
> (Male, blind, degenerative.)

> 'I felt terrible, very upset, always crying. I lost everything then.'

> 'I felt very upset at this time.'

> 'Lowering, my nerves have gone, they have been shattered by this (registration).'

> 'It felt like the end, something absolute.'
>
> (Female, 40–55, partially sighted.)

> 'I was crying day and night, wished I had not gone through with the operation in the first place.'

The intervention of a social worker working with the ophthalmologist throughout the period of registration, and being available at a specialist registration clinic, could identify those more in need of assistance, and respond accordingly. More disturbing and tragic consequences about the impact or registration were poignantly revealed by some of the individuals in this study:

> 'It just didn't sink in. A few days later I had a severe heart attack and I often wonder if it was stress of this (registration) and what I had been through.'
>
> (Female, blind, degenerative.)

> 'It was a great shock, my husband's death, then my loss of vision, it was all too much. I started drinking heavily.'

'Terrific shock. I was put on tranquillizers but later I said I think I can cope and came off them.'

'Shocked as so sudden, I had a heart attack soon after.'

(Female, blind, degenerative.)

Whilst the onset of coronary or physical illness was apparently attributed to the shock of registration, there is no telling whether or not registration was the culmination of other stressful factors; namely, for want of an ideal analogy, 'the straw that broke the camel's back'. Furthermore, there is no way of establishing whether such illness was part and parcel of the condition which initially undermined eye sight.

Emotional repercussions for the families involved were also highlighted:

'Numb, my wife was very shocked—she could not take it, as she had mental problems—four months later she committed suicide.'

'I felt very sorry for myself, I did not let my family know how bad I felt.'

'Registration!—got to be done, that's it, best to know these things—my family took it worse than I did.'

These extremes and tragic consequences are by no means isolated incidents within the study. These patients attributed loss of sight, and particularly the process of registration, with other major life crises. The above examples refer to addiction and suicide, which indicate the extent of distress caused, and hints at the unmet need to recognise the stress potentially involved. The following comments were fairly typical of just over a third of those in the study, who felt they needed emotional help and counselling when registered:

'If I had someone to talk with about my loss of sight, I would have appreciated psychological help to discuss emotional problems, such as anger and grief. Right now I feel I would still like and appreciate this help.'

'I wanted to talk about how I felt - how was I going to do normal things again?'

(Female, blind, degenerative.)

'I would have liked someone to come and talk to me about it all.'

(Female, partially sighted, degenerative.)

'Just to learn what was happening.'

It is suggested that extreme emotional distress, as revealed in the above quotations, may be diminished, or at least speedily identified and responded to, by counselling.

2. Stigmatization

Another striking area of concern for the group concerning registration was their sense of being labelled or stigmatized. The type of anxiety expressed varied in degree but seemed to suggest an underlying disquiet about being socially rejected because of the disability and being registered. It may be that such worries about becoming stigmatized are bound up with the individual's previous perceptions, experience and bias towards the disabled. A significant internal shift is called for in the process of losing a major sense such as sight, in that the attitudes and expectations held about the disabled begin to have personal relevance for the afflicted individual. How 'you', as an able-bodied person, judged the disabled will at some level affect the judgment of yourself as disabled, i.e. how 'you' view yourself in joining the ranks of the disabled (refer also to Chapter 6):

> 'I didn't want it, I wouldn't admit to being disabled. It is not a word that would fit in with my life. Instead of being one person, I was one of a group—I felt no one cared.'

> 'I saw myself as a classified cripple or something, someone with a disability.'

Other comments linked the concept of group identity with being spied on or controlled. Some spoke more broadly of general distaste in becoming registered. An impression which was emphasized was that they were not appropriately aware of the voluntary nature of registration:

> 'You are not free any more, they come and ask questions and want to know your whole pedigree.'

> 'Didn't want to be registered, found it dreadful, it made me feel depressed.'

> 'I did not like it at all, I thought it was awful.'

One gentleman expressed fear that registration could jeopardize his employment:

> 'At first I didn't want to know. I wanted to keep my job a little longer. On the other hand I could see some advantages.'

This study recommends that the voluntary nature of registration should be stressed by both the ophthalmologist and social worker who attends the disabled person enabling the client to exercise choice about whether or not they want to be registered. Such advice seems particularly useful when it is remembered that this and other studies have found that generally people did not seem to be aware of the voluntary nature of registration.

3. Negative Denial Response

One of the recurring issues that appeared striking was the sizable group of people who apparently tried to block off, shut out or deny any feelings whatsoever about loss of sight and registration. A very common response was of the type: 'tried not to think about it as it upset me too much.'

There was a sense in which some patients were attempting to screen off a level of emotion which was felt by them to be unacceptable. It was noted that amongst others in this category that a more neutral response was reported. This apparent neutrality appeared to be an absence of any emotion whatsoever, with a very common report being: 'had no feelings at all.'

Whilst in the early days such a response might be expected in conjunction with shock reaction, the seemingly chronic lack of emotion amongst those who were interviewed was felt to be curious. The following statements encapsulate the more typical response in this category:

> 'No, I just did not think of it. I am the sort of person who was always out and about, and what if I couldn't get out any more'

> 'I never really had any feelings about registration, there wasn't anything that could be done so it didn't make any difference to me.'

> 'Shut it out of mind.'

> (Male, blind, degenerative.)

The constancy of suppressed or denied affect will be explored in greater detail later in the book.

4. Resignation

Stoicism was expressed in connection with registration suggesting a level of acceptance and, in a few cases, an optimistic beginning.

In terms of what it means to be registered as blind or partially sighted, and the feelings associated with registration, typical replies in this category were:

> 'Nothing, that was that.'

> (Female, partially sighted, degenerative.)

> 'I have not really given any thought to it (registration).'

> (Female, blind.)

> 'I took it all calm, collected.'

> (Female, partially sighted, degenerative.)

> 'I did not take a lot of notice. I did not really know what it meant.'

> (Female, partially sighted, degenerative.)

> 'I didn't feel any different. It doesn't make any difference.'

> (Female, partially sighted, degenerative.)

'I didn't think anything, just accepted it as part of getting old.'

(Female, blind.)

A few patients within the study viewed becoming registered as visually impaired as a positive turning point; some spoke of optimism for the future, whilst others took a positively pragmatic view of registration, believing that there would be additional financial benefits from this process. The question of perceived advantages and disadvantages to registration will be explored later.

Only one person in the study actively asked to be registered as visually impaired. Her reflection conveyed this sense of tolerance and acceptance. When asked 'what did it mean to you to be registered as blind (or partially sighted)', this lady replied:

'Not much, as I had asked to be registered. I knew all blind people were registered. I thought "Well, if I am short sighted I should declare the fact that I can't see people." People move and let me sit down now; they behave more respectfully when they see a white stick.'

(Female, partially sighted, degenerative.)

One lady commented somewhat ambiguously, and perhaps concernedly, that she felt being registered was 'hope for improvement' (female, blind, degenerative).

Such a comment, whilst optimistic in character, might also hint at unrealistic hope for visual improvement as opposed to improvement in services. Others viewed registration as providing access to much needed supervision and support. Three people saw registration as positively singling them out for special attention:

'Only that I was under somebody's supervision and being looked after.'
'Just meant that there were social people you could get in touch with. You are handicapped.'

One of these seemed to feel that registration would entitle them to alternative medical assistance than would be available if they had remained unregistered:

'All it meant to me was that I would get better treatment for my sight.'

Preparation for registration

Many patients reported being totally unprepared for registration. Earlier in this section acute psycho-social distress was discussed. These two factors, unpreparedness for registration and acute psychological distress, appear to be interrelated. It is recalled that just under a third of all those interviewed (31) felt that their doctor had not helped them prepare for loss of sight. It is to be expected therefore that they would not have been able to prepare for the implications of registration. This sense of unpreparedness was reflected in numerous replies:

> 'Did not prepare at all for my sight loss.'
>
> (Female, partially sighted, degenerative.)

> 'I was not able to prepare, it was a big shock.'

It was also noticed that a couple of people had difficulties with emotional preparation despite the gradual onset and deterioration of their loss of sight. This would seem to support our contention that for some patients forewarning of visual loss is not in itself an adequate preparation for the changes loss of sight will bring:

> 'It happened over two years but I was not able to prepare fully.'

> 'I was not prepared to see myself as a registered person.'
>
> (Female, blind, degenerative.)

Throughout this book consideration has focused on what factors might help or hinder the patients at every stage of their career in disability in emotionally and practically preparing for loss of sight and registration. From the testimonies offered by individuals in each of the groups discussed above, the following points were noted. First, patients are not aware that they are being registered and potentially not adequately aware of the voluntary nature of registration, the implications for it and the services available. It is suggested that such hazy or vague notions about registration will leave patients potentially unprepared when the time comes to be registered—a time when they are emotionally more vulnerable, uncertain and afraid about what the future holds for them. They should specifically be told what assistance they are going to be given by the doctor and social worker to aid them in facing up to the changes of living with visual impairment.

Second, we asked how the future following registration was perceived. A common response was a form of negative denial which seemed to go one step further than just denying the loss of vision, moving on to deny any feelings which may have been associated with the loss. If one denies the reality of a major life change then by implication one has to simultaneously deny any feelings that might be associated with that stress. These responses outweighed other sorts of replies concerning perceptions of the future:

> 'Never thought about it. Looking ahead had never been one of my things. I was not going to start then thinking about the future.'

> 'I just felt I would go on as usual whether I liked it or not.'
>
> (Female, blind, degenerative.)

> 'Just have to live with it, have no choice.'
>
> (Male, partially sighted, degenerative.)

'Have to grin and bear it.'

(Male, blind, degenerative.)

'I didn't and don't think of the future now.'

(Female, blind, trauma.)

The second most significant set of replies gathered from qualitative statements about their view of the future showed feelings of despair, helplessness, depression and frustration. It is worth stressing that this question was asked in the past tense, but that many of them chose to answer in the present tense, perhaps suggesting that the feelings they had about the future at the time of registration were still troubling them up to two years later. This supposition suggests that without particular types of help clients' perceptions of the future and their role in exercising choice and carving out a life for themselves may remain unaltered over time. A typical selection of quotations for those people in this second group are give below:

'I live day to day.'

(Female, blind, degenerative.)

'I take one day at a time.'

This type of response, although not unusual in response to crisis, may suggest an unwillingness to face the future—a symptom of chronic depression. Within the counselling contract an assessment is made of the client's ability to project thoughts forward and to plan or to orientate a new life style. Therefore, the above comments might be construed as exhibiting a level of depression which the client may not have consciously registered:

'I see the future as a downward road.'

Another interesting element in some of these replies is the poignant and often symbolic choice of words used to describe internal perceptions and feelings about visual loss. For example:

'I see the future as very bleak, very dark.'

'I saw, and see, no future.'

(Male, partially sighted, degenerative.)

'Very bleak.'

(Female, partially sighted, degenerative.)

'There is nothing but blackness inside me.'

Such descriptions may illustrate a physical reality, but they also symbolize an internal expression of emotional disquiet (refer also to the case example of Mary in Chapter 7).

Perceived advantages of registration

Generally speaking the patients in this study attributed practical advantages to registration. There was a general expectation that more money and financial benefits would be forthcoming as a consequence of becoming registered, and in a couple of instances frustration was expressed when aspirations were not met:

'More money. I thought I might get a bit more.'

'Only £1.25 a week, that's all.'

'Attendance allowance, financial help.'

'Thought might get financial help.'

'Financial benefits, and there were none. I had the wrong idea. A great disappointment financially. I thought it would solve some, if not all of my problems.'

(Male, blind, degenerative.)

Other commonly reported advantages were seen as practical aid to daily living, rehabilitation services and advice giving:

'Practical help and advice.'

'The doctor said I would get a talking book and help and advice.'

As previously mentioned in this chapter, it was noted that several patients seemed to have hazy and unclear ideas about the range of services available following registration. A sizable proportion, over one-third of the group, said they could not comment on any advantages, as they were aware of none. Vagueness concerning perceived advantages was summed up in the comment made by one woman:

'I would probably have facilities that a blind person would be entitled to, but I am not sure what these are.'

Several felt the main advantage of being registered was the receipt of a talking book. Another perceived advantage mentioned by several in the group was the sense that registration was a safeguard against neglect or rejection by professional services:

'Not being rejected after the hospital could do no more for me.'

(Female, blind, degenerative.)

'Somebody there.'

(Female, partially sighted, trauma.)

That clients need to feel supported and reassured about the range of services available to them is understandable at a time of potential stress and uncertainty. As we shall see later in this chapter, it is important that unnecessary delays within the process of the registration should be kept to a minimum and that clients are seen as soon as possible by a social worker following registration, in order that they may share their feelings about this situation and raise any questions or doubts they have.

One gentleman defined the main advantage to registration as being a declaration of the fact that he could not see. Only one person cited registration as being of positive benefit to obtain employment. Only three people in the study were in employment.

> 'Didn't see any advantages except thought might get help for getting work.'

Perceived disadvantages of registration

Despite the fact that several people had earlier reported that they could not see any particular advantages of registration, most equally claimed they could see no disadvantages. A typical comment was:

> 'Not really, because you don't lose out on it, do you?'

Several said that registration did not really make any difference to them either way and therefore there were no particular comments to be made strongly in either direction. One might question the effectiveness of a system where the recipients express indifference and are unable to define any clear advantages or disadvantages. If the process of registration was attaining the aims which had been put forward for its implementation, namely, to promote the welfare of the visually impaired population, then registrants should be able to effectively evaluate the pros and cons of registration as befits their individual needs.

It is perhaps hopeful that even if registration is not automatically seen as advantageous by recipients, equally it is not detrimental: it does no harm and serves, as results show, to support some individuals who feel protected and supervised within the community. We must constructively ensure that such supervision and assistance is a reality of the registration system.

Time taken to complete the registration process

There are three distinct administrative phases entailed in registration prior to the client being assessed for rehabilitative services. The study explored the time it took for each of these stages to be completed as it was strongly felt that the time factor was an important element in the client's career. Where possible, information gathered from patients was cross checked with hospital and social services records concerning the processing of BD8 forms.

The stages involved in the process of registration are:

1. From ophthalmic examination for eligibility to completion of BD8 forms

2. Certification of BD8 forms and time between receipt in social services departments

3. From receipt of BD8 forms in social services to first contact with client.

In Stage One only 39 people could recall the time between the last examination with their ophthalmologist before the recorded completion of BD8 forms. Of these, thirteen said it was within a week, nine recalled discussion within six months, and one within the first year. It may be surmised from these limited findings that once registration is felt to be appropriate by the ophthalmologist, registration is carried through without undue delay, possibly at the next three or six month clinic review. However, the most notable delays appear during Stage Two, seeming to arise out of the completion of BD8 forms following examination and the actual receipt of them in social services departments.

Out of the 79 patients who gave information, 43 had to wait up to three months for the registration papers (form BD8) to be processed through to their local social services departments. Five were delayed up to six months following examination, with one unfortunate patient waiting up to one year for the social services to receive form BD8. Many factors could account for this delay. For example, the pressure on ophthalmologists in completing BD8 forms once patients have been seen in busy clinics, and the scarcity of secretarial and administrative support to process completed forms. It cannot be established whether such pressures and staff shortages account for delays at the hospital end, but the sheer number of patients attending large centralized clinics may also contribute to this process. It is clear that unnecessary delay forestalls vital rehabilitation and entitlement to benefits and services that patients require.

It may be hypothesised that a delay at the hospital end of the process makes it evident that there is a need for an increase in medical and nursing personnel to care for these patients, and also for adequate administrative staff to ensure the efficient processing of the paperwork involved. It is recommended that emphasis be placed on the importance of facilitating early and speedy registration.

It would have been interesting to document time delays at each stage of the registration process. However, information was not available concerning the time BD8 forms were received within the local authority (Stage Three) and processed through to local area social services departments. Whilst patients felt that once BD8 forms were received in respective social services departments they were visited relatively quickly, in reality 46 had to wait up to three months for a visit, with 14 patients waiting anything between six months and one year for contact (see Table 5.2).

The wait for a visit was longer in Authority 'B', with 26 patients waiting up to three months, as opposed to 17 in Authority 'A'.

It is important to bear in mind that if patients are unaware in the first place that they have been registered as visually impaired, they are not in an

Table 5.2 How long after registration did the social worker visit?

	Number	Percentage
Within three months	46	45%
Within six months	10	9%
Within one year	4	4%
Not at all	1	1%
Can't remember	25	24%
No answer	18	17%

informed position to ask for assistance. Furthermore, loss of vision tends to affect the majority in middle to late years, and this group is arguably less vocal in asserting their needs and asserting their rights.

On a more positive note, 13 people had been visited prior to registration itself. Of these, five received help up to one year before certification as visually impaired. Such preventative practice on the part of social workers is to be commended. It potentially forestalls greater problems at a later stage for the client. Further research into the adjustment of those patients who had been given prophylactic assistance before significant sight loss has occurred might prove valuable. It might be argued that acquiring such skills as braille and stick assisted mobility can be enhanced if taught while there is useful remaining vision.

It is suggested that the process of registration itself may come too late in the day for some patients when at the time of registration they have lost a significant amount of vision.

The study recommends that entitlement of assistance and services should not be dependent upon the process of registration, which as we have seen in this chapter is potentially prone to delays and mishaps.

Summary and recommendations

One of the questions posed by this study was whether patients were being given a clear explanation of the purpose or implications of registration. Just under half the patients in this study (48%) discussed registration with the ophthalmologist. However, over a third of the group claimed they did not discuss registration with either hospital doctor or nurse. This group discussed registration with a specialist worker at home following registration and therefore did not have the opportunity to exercise choice about whether or not they wished to become registered as visually impaired.

It is a matter of concern that nine patients had to wait a year following diagnosis before registration was discussed. Whilst it is accepted that many patients might have been attending the hospital before they became eligible for registration as visually impaired, and that the delay between disclosure of diagnosis and discussion of registration might also have been dependent on medical investigations to establish the extent or permanency of visual damage, it is disquieting that 11 patients stated that registration had never been discussed with them at any stage although they were all subsequently registered. Eight in this group were registered as partially sighted which might imply an underestimation of the social and emotional upheaval that partial sight may evoke.

There is a tendency for registration to be discussed sooner with blind patients than with their partially sighted peers. Just over a third of the group found the discussion concerning registration adequate; of these a large proportion were blind. It is noted that just under a quarter reported that discussion of registration had been inadequate, but this did not appear to be significantly related to the extent of sight loss. Rather it reflected that too little information was given about the purpose for registration, as previously discussed in this chapter.

The assessment of patients' emotional response to registration suggested that acute psycho-social distress constituted the commonest recurring theme of all replies. Some attributed registration as being the cause of coronary heart attacks, physical illness and, in one tragic incident, prompting the suicide of a family member. Over a third of the patients interviewed said they would have welcomed counselling at this stage. Stigmatisation was another concern high on the patients' list as a possible disadvantage in becoming registered.

It is noted that the voluntary nature of registration seemed little emphasised to potential registrants, and there was a sense in which some felt resigned and powerless on becoming registered.

An interesting aspect of this investigation is that several reported an absence of any feelings whatsoever. However, for all other responses it was repeatedly asserted that patients were in no way prepared for becoming registered as visually impaired. There was a tendency for some patients to choose uncannily emotive and pertinent adjectives in describing their internal psychological state and their perception of the future.

Recommendations

1. That the provision of prior rehabilitative training from social service departments should not be dependent upon registration as visually impaired.

2. The voluntary nature of registration should be stressed to the affected individuals and their families at every stage of the registration.

3. The involvement of a specialist social worker working with the consultant ophthalmologist during specialist registration clinics would provide early assessment and prioritization of those most in need of practical and emotional assistance in adjusting to registration.

4. Greater collaboration between hospital based consultant ophthalmologists and area social workers would promote the likelihood that no patients would leave hospital unaware that they had been registered, facilitating earlier assistance and overriding bureaucratic procedures.

5. Additional administrative support in hospital based services might facilitate earlier completion of BD8 forms.

6. Further comparative research of clients who have received prophylactic assistance prior to registration and those experiencing delayed assistance might prove fruitful.

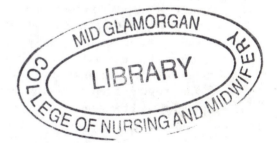

Chapter 6

What Does The Future Hold Now?
Patients' Psycho-Social Response to Loss of Vision

Introduction

The quest to explore the 'whole person' response to the change and potential crisis of deteriorating vision forms the core of this chapter, and indeed the cornerstone of this book. The immensity and complexity of such a task is testified by the almost infinite variety and uniqueness of individuals. The study tackled the problem by devising a multi-faceted assessment of personality predisposition and response. The intellectual, emotional, social, behavioural, philosophical, and health factors of patients were considered.[1] The interview questions that form the basis of this section evolved out of the typical comments received earlier from individuals facing major loss or change because of chronic disability. The patients in the group were asked to concur with or refute descriptive statements as being relevant to their experience at three stages:

(a) before loss of sight;

(b) at time of loss or deterioration; and

(c) when interviewed up to two years later.

These statements could be defined as experimental adjectives and were arranged for consideration in the following way.

1. *Practical*—relating to issues of practical daily living, coping around the house, domestic chores, care of self, mobility, financial planning, occupation and training and leisure pursuits.

2. *Physical/Health*—exploring self-care, addictive tendencies, physical response or illness following loss of sight and disruptive sleep patterns, etc.

3. *Worry, anxiety, pain, puzzlement*—exploring the range and intensity of emotional response, affecting every aspect of functioning and lifestyle.

4. *Denial, despair, anger, bitterness and refusal*—(refer also to the Appendix for categorization of questions). Possibly one of the most important

---

[1] Adapted from the London Hospital Bereavement Service Model of Counselling.

sections in the studying, exploring intense emotional response; denial and rejection following impairment, feelings of futility and despair, the instance of suicidal tendencies and attempts.

5. *Self-image*—considering self-esteem, fantasies about others percep-tions of disability, notions about self-worth and subsequent interac-tion with others.

6. *Worries about relationships with others*—elucidating issues concerning social stigmatization and the subsequent response of the affected individual, uncertain or ambivalent social interactions, and shame about disability.

7. *Negative changes in social relationships*—explorating primary relation-ships, with family and friends, and stereotypes concerning disability, etc.

Although categorized for convenience these areas of response are interde-pendent and overlapping. Any major change is rather like throwing a pebble into a pond; it is not just the splash of the stone hitting the water which is recorded, but the ripples throughout the pond which affect every part of its surface. Loss of sight or other disability, although superficially affecting one part of the body or physical sense, has ripple effects throughout the whole person and his or her social network. Only a modest reflection of the complexity of all these factors constantly interchanging and impinging upon one another may be realistically possible.

Before commencing the holistic section which forms the second part of this chapter, it is necessary to explore the extent to which notions about disability and visual impairment previously held by the group affected them after sight loss. Issues concerning negative denial, which was briefly eluci-dated in Chapter 5, and some relevant case examples will be considered. Exploring different interpretations and responses the health/care worker may make in response to this denial is central to extend the thinking and discussion contained in Chapter 7 and bring to life the nature of the coun-selling relationship. By questioning what professional care-givers choose to tune into and selectively hear or ignore, the opportunity to extend and enhance professional practice is advanced. It is hoped that the examples in this first section will promote professional development, at least provoking thought and discussion about various alternative interventions at different stages of the client's career.

For social workers, the training ethos has been to adopt a problem solving strategy. Arguably such a philosophy may lead to a distorted assessment of the client's capabilities, overlooking their potential for self-improvement and growth out of crisis. From 'grief to growth' is a wise maxim: experience has shown time and time again that major life crises can provoke new depths of self-insight, personal growth and development which may have lain untapped but for the dynamic stress of change. Under pressure, individuals may bring forth qualities which had hitherto lain dormant. Therefore, whilst the assessment of the holistic categories will consider the negative and distressing side of change, specifically exploring where vulnerability lies, this is intended only to highlight areas of need where care workers may make effective contributions and interventions and help clients to identify these potential 'sore spots'. There is equally a need to explore the incidence of improvement or positive change brought about by the crisis of loss of sight. In this way the study hopes to retain as far as possible a sense of realistic balance between needs that are not met and the strong coping elements within all of us. To question what circumstances or qualities allow one human being to cope better than another is virtually an impossible task. However, to tentatively identify those clients who have appeared to fare better throughout their career in disability—physically, practically and emotionally—allows understanding about what sort of help might increase this likelihood for others.

The chapter will conclude with a brief summary and recommendations for practice.

Do we become what we think we are?
(Perceptions of visually impaired people)

In attempting to unravel the complexity of psychological and emotional response to loss of sight the question arises 'Do we become what we think we are?', or in other words, would one's former perceptions, experiences and possible prejudice of the disabled, and more particularly visually impaired people, affect in any way an individual's response to loss of sight? If so, in what way are these previous notions internalized and affect the disabled individual's perception of self? No longer is it a case of 'them and us'; the individual has joined the ranks of those previously respected, valued, patronized or rejected. Therefore the participants were asked what they thought about blind and partially sighted people before they lost their sight. The most common response was that they had pitied and felt sorry for blind people, some seeing them as pathetic objects:

'I always used to help. I felt sorry for them.'

(Male, partially sighted, degenerative.)

'I felt sick with worry in case they bashed into the wall or got run over.'

(Female, blind, degenerative.)

'I thought it was a dreadful thing.'

(Female, blind.)

'I have always seen partially sighted people as being sighted. I felt sorry for the blind. I felt they were in a different world.'

(Female, blind, degenerative.)

Notably, three of the above were themselves blind. There appeared to be a general tendency for those who had previously pitied visually impaired people not to really connect themselves with the situation and circumstances they described. Where connections were made, there was a sense in which any difficulty experienced was not relevant to them personally, but somehow was felt to be present for other people. Such a response might be psychoanalytically defined as projection, e.g. the problem was externally projected onto other disabled people and any discomfort felt by them is seen as located outside.

'I never thought my eyesight would go like this. I thought how terrible it was for other people.'

(Female, partially sighted, degenerative.)

'To be perfectly honest, I did not think much about it. It must be dreadful to be really blind.'

(Female, blind, degenerative.)

In other cases individuals spoke in the future tense, even though they had lost a substantial degree of sight. The hope that it would never happen to them indicates a perceived differentiation between themselves and disabled people.

'Hope it never happens to me.'

(Female, blind, degenerative.)

'I thought it was a terrible thing. When you look at people you think "Cor, I would not like to be like that".'

(Male, blind, degenerative.)

'I always prayed I would never go blind.'

(Female, partially sighted, degenerative.)

Of course, any remaining eye sight will be seen as a boon and even the smallest degree of light perception may be used to maximum effect. Many registered blind people are not totally blind in the stereotypical view of blindness, but have much useful remaining vision either for mobility or for reading with visual aids. Therefore, perhaps it is to be appreciated that it is a natural response not to perceive oneself as belonging to the group which is defined according to expectations and experiences, as blind or partially sighted. Equally such a response appears to be a subtle form of denial. Several people appeared to take their former brief encounters with the visually impaired population in their stride. Where there had been a previous positive perception of the disabled person it appeared that their own loss was tolerated that much more equably. It might be that previously held respect and admiration for disabled people will at some level suggest to the affected individual that they now will also be positively viewed by society and assisted without underlying patronage or prejudice.

'I often saw them. I marvelled at the way they got about. I was always told to wait until they asked for help, not to offer it. This kept their self-confidence up and has helped me.'

(Male, blind, degenerative.)

'I saw people with dogs. They were doing many things and getting about.'

(Male, blind, degenerative.)

'I didn't think about it. They were just people. I was always pleased to help them along.'

(Female, blind, degenerative.)

'Never gave them a thought. I would offer help to cross the road if they were waiting.'

(Female, blind, trauma.)

There were a few cases where families played an influential role in determining self-perception and social definition of the visually impaired. The experience of being reared by, or having, visually impaired siblings because of hereditary genetic factors had understandably influenced perceptions about visual difficulties.

'I never thought about it. We have had so much trouble with my son and his eyes, and my husband was always short-sighted, and had to have corneal grafts, I was used to it somehow.'

(Female, partially sighted, degenerative.)

Another gentleman appeared to have learnt a salient lesson from watching his father's misfortunes. He used this experience to adapt and amend his own response accordingly.

'My father was blind unfortunately. He refused all offers of help and blundered his way through just about everything. I was determined not to do this when I knew. Also father never talked about it!'

(Male, blind, degenerative.)

Overall what appeared to be significant about these replies was that whilst these patients were able both to positively connote and realistically define the difficulties and potentialities for visually impaired people (expressed in their memories about how they saw blind or partially sighted people before they lost their own sight), there was a prevailing sense of separateness from the group they sought to define. Whilst we might tentatively question whether this is a subtle form of protective denial as a defence mechanism, it is equally unclear whether previously held negative views of visual handicap impinged on the affected individual's psyche and response to this change. Those who had held previously positive notions about visual handicap felt they had adjusted better.

Case examples and alternatives for practice

There are two specific and potentially sensitive emotional responses which the client may manifest following loss of sight. Negative denial may be one such response which forces the individual to push away or reject the reality of his visual impairment and subsequently deny any emotions or responses which might normally be anticipated. The second example refers to suicidal tendency, which is itself something of a social taboo and consequently may engender in the inexperienced worker unconscious or conscious feelings of discomfort, fearing to focus on the client's vulnerability. We will explore the various responses that the care worker, whether doctor, nurse or social worker, may make in relation to these two situations. The social worker who, seeing the client in the security of their own home, with greater opportunity of time, may have the potential for exploring such issues in depth.

The worker who has given some thought to his or her own emotional vulnerability and physical mortality and who has had the opportunity to explore his or her own feelings in relation to life crisis, death and suicide, will be potentially more at ease and in control when exploring these areas with the client. If we are more aware of our own resistances and defences these are less likely to get in the way of our work with clients.

Negative denial

For the purpose of this book negative denial refers to the mechanism by which an individual may suppress, deny or block out the painful areas of reality and in consequence have to sublimate any affect, emotion or action which reinforces the reality (in this case loss of sight) which he or she seeks to deny. The destructiveness of this circular double bind is all too clear and may be seen at various stages in the affected individual's career in disability. Such a response might not be constant but may fluctuate in response to other factors. Certainly in the early stages of loss, shock, denial and anger are common, natural and potentially healthy self-protecting mechanisms. Negative denial suggests a longer-term and more entrenched chronic response which becomes self-limiting and restrictive. The professional worker should seek to detect its presence and work through such a response with the client.

Let us assume that the client in these two case examples has requested counselling. Indeed, no counselling should be initiated unless the client has requested it and is motivated to undertake such work. All too often well-intentioned professionals may suggest to the patient that it would help to talk to somebody and intimate that the help offered covers a whole range of practical services as well. In such instances the client may be confused about why he or she is meeting the counsellor and may have different expectations about the purpose of the interchange. It is advisable to sensitively but unambiguously share with the patient or client the feelings that he or she might benefit from counselling, outlining what this entails before referral on to a counsellor or therapist. This prepares clients and allows them to gauge whether or not they wish to participate in counselling, and it acts as a healthy starting point for more effective intervention. In the examples that follow (see Tables 6.1 and 6.2) the interpretation which may be put on clients' statements to explain the relevance of the worker's response is considered. This is not to suggest, however, that there is ever only one interpretation to be made. In utilising theory in practice one needs to hypothesize from the total interaction with the client, assessing non-verbal behaviour, voice intimation, your feelings in relation to him or her, i.e. counter-transference, and what unacknowledged feelings and responses may underlie certain statements. It is unacceptable arrogance in any worker to assume that there is only one explanation or interpretation of behaviour and material. Any hypothesis of why a client is showing a particular effect or response has to be taken within the total context of (a) assessment, (b) the particular session in question, and (c) other relevant knowledge (from liaison with other rehabilitation workers etc.) In these examples the more common sorts of statements made by clients will be presented, linked to interpretations which were found to be facilitating and helpful in appropriately directing the clients' response.

Obviously such an extract constitutes only a minor part of one session within the overall counselling contract and should be viewed in that context. It is important not to confuse Linderman's categorizations of reaction to grief; of pure denial with negative denial. Linderman and others suggest that denial is expressed by the inability to accept the loss, occasionally resulting in absolute denial. Negative denial appears by contrast to assume a more chronic low-key aspect, trivializing or downgrading the impact and extent about what has happened. Such a response appears to result in greater intolerance, impatience and warding off of consequent grief than might be normally expected. Many factors may account for this often unacknowledged reaction; fear of 'letting go', losing control and being overwhelmed by one's feelings; embarrassment or guilt in having certain emotions; and anger, which seems especially hard to own.

Social expectations and taboos undoubtedly bolster such reservations. In the West we culturally appear to condone 'the stiff upper lip tradition' with the familiar refrain 'wasn't he/she brave' arising from potentially painful situations. It should not be surprising that such subtle defences used on a massive scale have more sinister and elusive repercussions for the individual under stress.

Table 6.1 Case example one

Client's Statement	Interpretation	Worker's response
1) 'Don't have any feelings, what's the point, I can't do anything about it.'	Suppression of emotion, query underlying despair/frustration/anger which could be turned in on the self later as depression.	1) 'It sounds like you're saying no use crying over spilt milk because you can't change what is happening to you.'
2) 'Yes, that's it, what's to be done?'	a) Establishment of empathy/rapport b) Positively connote client's view of strength, avoid critical statements. c) Give permission to own powerful feelings.	2)(a) 'That's a determined and philosophical outlook which is good to hold on to. In my experience though it is common for people facing loss of sight, like yourself, to feel frustrated about what is happening and so try to push it from their minds, not to think about it.' b) 'A lot of people would have been angry at a time like this. What have been some of your feelings?'
3) 'Well, I try not to think about how I am, I don't want to get upset.'	Some shift in admitting cause for dis-ease.	3) 'You are saying if you think about it, you get upset?' (feel low/sad/ miserable/down).
4) 'Yes, I suppose so.'		4) 'What sort of things upset you?'
5) 'Oh, I don't know, seeing Jim, my husband, choked up or my bumping into things.'	Equilibrium through avoidance is disrupted by demonstration of others' distress or a major change in functioning is underlined by a domestic accident which reinforcers eality of sight loss.	5)(a) 'You feel uncomfortable when your family is upset? What do you do/or say then?' b) 'How are you able to express your feelings at these times?'
6) 'I try to change the subject, or laugh it off. Doesn't do to get upset, best thing for everyone not to talk about it.	Query family collusion against emotional pain of grief. N.B. In assessing the extent of family collusion with negative denial one might ask 'Who is most/least upset in the family about what has happened.'	6)(a) 'It sounds like you might be afraid about what will happen if you were to talk about your loss of sight? (b) 'What do you think would happen if you were to share with your family what you feel now?'
7) 'Hmm, well I don't want to get upset.'	Permission to grieve.	7) 'How do you express your sadness about what has happened to you? What do you do to show you are upset? What do you do/say to show you are unhappy/ sad?'

Client's Statement	Interpretation	Worker's response
8) 'Not sure really, never thought about it much before, guess I go into myself, think about it a lot at night, sometimes I cry when I am alone, all sorts of things going through my mind then'.	Acknowledgement of range of emotions, greater insight into response, potentially heralding beginning of movement forward to look at broader issues of response and adjustment.	8)(a) 'You are saying all sorts of worries and thought go through your head. What worries you most about losing your sight?' (b) 'Thoughts going round and round inside can be very upsetting. What troubles you most?'
9) 'How am I going to manage—I can't always pretend not to care, Don't want family to have to do everything for me.'	Great tolerance of emotional and broader needs.	9) 'I know it's never easy to about feelings, you have been honest and open which will help us explore how to tolerate what has happened to you and make new plans for the future.'

Suicidal tendencies

Suicide risk must always be assessed when counselling an individual who has suffered major permanent physical disability. Any clues or leads that the client gives must be picked up and responded to. It is imperative that suicidal risk be constantly re-evaluated and assessed throughout the whole of the counselling contract. It may be necessary to confront implied suicidal tendencies. Whilst raising the issue of suicide does not itself decrease the risk of an attempt, equally the myth that talking about suicide increases its likelihood because of suggestion is unfounded. Therefore, as previously mentioned, it is helpful for the counsellor to reflect on his or her own attitudes and/or experiences in relation to suicide.

One of the most startling and significant findings of this project was the continually high incidence of suicidal thoughts linked to intense feelings of despair and futility of life. Twenty four patients[2] reported that they had no hope for the future, both at the time of loss and when interviewed two years later. Of the total group, twelve reported feeling that the meaning had left life during their loss of sight. This number rose to 21 who felt the meaning had left life only since the loss. In addition, 20 patients reported feeling their world had crumbled at time of loss, with 16 experiencing this distressing response up to two years following loss of sight.

Out of the complete group, 21 reported thinking of taking their own lives at some point in their career in disability, with four people asserting that they still felt suicidal. Tragically, 13 people within the group had made an attempt on their lives; of these, only one had attempted suicide prior to loss. One distressed individual felt when interviewed that this was still a possibility.

---

[2] All the above material was derived from the total group.

The seriousness and potential tragedy of these results speak for themselves, demonstrating that to avoid discussion of suicide does not make the problem go away. One courageous but distressed lady was able to expose for the first time during the interview that she had previously made three former attempts on her life which had been misconstrued as accidents by other family members. The interview gave her an opportunity to own what was for her a devastating reality and expression of the distress caused by loss of sight. Whilst this is an extreme situation, it serves to demonstrate that there is potentially a need which is not met for this particular client group. As professional care workers, we all share a duty to sensitively address and confront the potentiality of suicide.

There are, broadly speaking, three distinct phases in the assessment of suicide risk[3]

Phase One—Assess whether suicide is intended or constitutes fantasy, i.e. is there a plan—when, where and how might this be executed? Does the client have the means? Is there any history of previous suicide attempts? In what ways were these attempts enacted? How might physical disability help or hinder any attempt?

Phase Two—The counsellor should be sensitively directive, express knowledge and rationalize suicide as one alternative when confronted with extreme stress and change. Encourage the client to make a commitment with regard to not attempting suicide. Facilitate and allow the client to feel responsible for his or her own actions and decisions. It is important to balance positive elements with negative, i.e. facilitate planning and hope for the future.

Phase Three—Assess risk to client of suicide, focus on professional responsibilities for instigating an alternative course of action: (a) referral to general practitioner, (b) request psychiatric opinion/hospitalization, (c) rehabilitation and counselling as appropriate.

How might the counsellor sensitively facilitate and explore this delicate issue?

The purpose of these examples is not to suggest that the ultimate aim of counselling should be to assail people's natural defences, but rather to tune into what might lie behind a certain statement: listening with an inner ear to what is being implied but left unsaid, and facilitating the client's ventilation of whatever concerns him or her.

There is a vast dichotomy between giving clients permission to grieve or to own powerful feelings which may have previously worried them ('Am I going mad?' syndrome), and inappropriately reducing them to tears or assailing their defence mechanisms. Professional integrity and respect for

---

[3] Phases of assessment adapted from the London Hospital Bereavement Service Model (1988).

Table 6.2. Case example one

Client's Statement	Intervention/ Intereation.	Counsellor's response
		General exploratory open ended question: 'What kind of feelings has losing your sight brought up for you?'
'So many thoughts. . . I feel empty inside some-times. I think what's the point of getting up. I'm not always sure how much more I can take.'	Sense of underlying futility, nothing to get up for/or go on for = query. It is less common for someone to come straight out and admit their 'plan'. They may not be sure of your reac-tion/judgement of them. The client needs to know you are able to talk about this possibility—so, it feels right, open up the topic.	a) 'Can you say a bit more abouth that?' OR b) 'When you are feeling esp-ecially low, does it get so bad it get so bad that you feel like ending it all?' OR c) 'Do you ever get so sad that you feel you can't go on any more, just don't want to live?' OR d) 'It's not at all unusual for people in your situation to feel, at times, like taking your life. Has that thought ever crossed your mind?'

one's client will ensure that the aims of counselling are uppermost when augmenting the counselling intervention[4]

The psychological and social reaction to loss of sight

It will be remembered that the adjustment dimensions relate to three stages in the client's experience:

(a) before loss of sight;

(b) at time of loss or deterioration; and

(c) when interviewed up to two years later.

Practical adjustment

As will be seen later, one of the surprises in this study was the fact that, overall, practical adjustment appeared to be less of a problem for the majority of people than achieving psychological and emotional tolerance of their visual handicap. Visual impairment, however, calls for numerous practical adjustments or adaptations to one's lifestyle. Within the practical category seven clients appeared to experience significant difficulty and

---

[4] The technique examples given above do not constitute a manual of counselling practice and should not be viewed or utilised in that light. The examples form only the minutest part of the overall practice and intervention of counselling.

deterioration following loss of sight[5]. As might be expected, the two areas of greatest difficulty were getting around alone and looking after the home. Forty-five clients reported deterioration in mobility and 31 found difficulty in looking after their homes. Only one person reported improvement at the time of interview in relation to these areas. A more subtle and perhaps more surprising concern was that 23 people expressed deterioration in their ability to make friends following their loss of sight and at the time of interview. Many factors could account for this situation; reticence on the part of the disabled person, embarrassment on both sides, people being unsure how to approach the disabled person or to open up and initiate discussion and friendship. Furthermore, sight is an essential part of non-verbal communication; making eye contact across a crowded room to hail an acquaintance. Also, reduced vision impedes mobility within a social gathering. For example, the visually impaired person becomes more reliant on others to introduce themselves, or to be taken across a crowded room. Thus the subtleties of socializing may be undermined. Loss of vision may also deny the disabled person the choice of who to talk with or who to avoid. It is spontaneity in social interaction which can be undermined by visual impairment. The consequence may be greater social isolation. However, it serves to underline the issue of social isolation as a consequence of physical disability. Fifteen patients felt that choice of friendships had been taken from them as a consequence of their visual impairment, whilst another 13 commented that one of the consequences of loss of sight was that others organized their lives. Both these groups, up to two years later, felt there had been no positive change in these areas. It is not easy to speculate about the possible causes for these particular circumstances, but whilst no strong claims are made, it might perhaps indicate that practical orientation and rehabilitation need to include in their curriculum some kind of assertiveness training to increase the level of self-determination for the disabled person. Given the emphasis on mobility training and practical rehabilitation, there appears to be a low level of improvement in relation to practical adjustment and daily living skills. It might have been surmised that at the time of interview two years later, patients would show a marked improvement in these areas. The study found that only one person reported improvement in personal care and mobility. The only other indicator of improvement was one lady who felt it was easier to make friends.

If, as the findings of this study seem to suggest, there is no or little improvement in daily living and mobility skills throughout a two year period, when presumably rehabilitation should have been provided, then we may reasonably ask whether or not such specialist services are appropriately targeted to achieve the overall aims of rehabilitation in the broadest sense (see Table 6.3).

---

[5] Please refer to the Appendix for categorization of adjustment dimensions.

Table 6.3. Practical dimension

Practical dimension	Number out of total group (Base Line 104)	
	Incidence of improvement since loss of sight	Incidence of deterioration since loss of sight and when interviewed
Difficulty looking after home	1	31
Difficulty taking care of myself	1	19
Worry about financial situation	1	17
Difficulty getting around alone	1	45
Problems with accommodation	-	9
Problems with job/studies	-	6
What was offered did not suit individual needs	-	9
Difficult to make friends	1	23
Not achieving potential	-	17
Others organised my life	-	-
Choice taken from my hand	-	15

Physical health

Preventative health care appears to have assumed much greater public importance within the last two decades. It may be suggested that increased stress and change brought about by sight loss might well undermine or affect the individual's health and general well being. Not surprisingly 11 people reported becoming ill following loss of sight, with only one reporting an improvement at the time of interview. It is a sobering thought that ten people remained in poor general health up to the time of interview. As the majority of our patients were over 50 years of age, perhaps this can be attributed to general deterioration caused by the ageing process. However, 13 reported having no energy following loss of sight, with improvement in only two cases. Lethargy and diminished energy could be an indicator of a level of depression, and in this connection ten of the interviewed group also felt that their general physical health had deteriorated following sight deterioration. In hindsight it is regrettable that this study did not have the resources and authority to verify this from general practitioner records because of confidentiality. Visual deterioration appears to have undermined the overall physical health of ten patients; they reported never feeling well following loss of sight. Improvement was reported in only three cases.

One lady reported drinking more as an immediate consequence of loss of sight, but at time of interview this reaction had diminished.

More concerningly, ten people reported an increase in their smoking consumption following loss of sight, with no apparent improvement over the two year period. No one reported lower consumption at interview. Another concerning factor in this area was that seven in the interview group reported taking sedatives as a result of loss of sight with again no diminishment or improvement when interviewed. Such a finding might support the contention that emotional and psychological help in the form of counselling may, for some individuals, replace the need for tranquillizers or anti- depressants which in essence only masks, or dampens, the emotional effect of the response to the crisis (see Table 6.4).

Table 6.4. Medical/health dimension

Medical/health dimension	Number out of total group (Base Line 104)	
	Incidence of improvement since loss of sight	Incidence of deterioration since loss of sight and when interviewed
Became ill	1	11
Had no energy	2	13
Never felt healthy	3	10
Drank more	1	1
Smoked more	-	10
Took sedatives	-	-

More recently the addictive properties of sedatives generally has been highlighted by the media and press. Such contemporary insight might explain the experiences of the patients in this study.

Worry, anxiety, emotional pain, puzzlement

The most interesting finding of this section was that overall there seemed to be a far greater incidence of deterioration than of subsequent improvement, not only at the time of loss, but following it. One of the highest levels of deterioration concerned attempts not to think about the loss. Just over a third of the group, 35 patients, reported trying not to think of sight loss. This would seem to have relevance to our earlier comments concerning negative denial. The second largest group in this section, 29 patients, reported deterioration in respect of worries about further changes that sight loss could bring. One gentleman reported improvement in this area between losing his sight and when interviewed. Similarly, of the 28 patients who reported feeling more vulnerable since sight loss, only two reported subsequent improvement at interview. Just under a quarter of the group (25) reported being unable to talk honestly about their worries. Only one individual felt there had been improvement in this area when interviewed. It appeared that patients felt they had 'to be strong' for others, and they felt that to talk honestly about their feelings might undermine the brave face that appeared to them to be necessary. Sixteen people felt worried most the time and said this was still an on-going problem. People were unable to talk about their inner feelings, were generally stressed and worried for a considerable time after sight loss and felt vulnerable or tried not to think about what had happened. It was noted that whilst coping with such reactions a sizable group felt unable to talk to others about their most pressing concerns. What does this say about the help of professionals involved in supporting patients and their family through these changes?

Whilst it is encouraging that a quarter of the group reported minimal disruption in issues concerning worry, anxiety, emotional pain and puzzlement, with a further 45 people experiencing between 10 and 50 percent of the list responses, it might be said that even if only one or two elements of concern or worry are experienced, this is enough to affect one's overall equilibrium and sense of wellbeing. Nineteen patients showed deterioration in between 50 and 100 percent of all the variables in this section, and it may be assumed that these individuals experienced severe emotional anxiety and worry (see Table 6.5).

Table 6.5. Worry, anxiety, emotional, pain, puzzlement

Worry, anxiety, emotional, pain, puzzlement	Number out of total group (Base Line 104)	
	Incidence of improvement since loss of sight	Incidence of deterioration since loss of sight and when interviewed
Lot of other worries, stresses	-	16
Examine philosophy of life (despair etc.)	-	10
Could not talk honestly about my worries	1	25
Felt vulnerable	2	28
Felt worried most of the time	3	16
Had mixed feelings	1	22
Questions have brought back painful memories	1	10
Worried about changes it would bring	1	29
Tried not to think of it	2	35
Not expect this at my age	3	25

Denial, despair, anger, bitterness, refusal to accept

This section, which is perhaps the most profoundly revealing of all the sections in the holistic assessment, demonstrated a high incidence of difficulty. Half reported experiencing some difficulty in 10 to 15 percent of the issues included in this category, and 18 experienced severe difficulty, with between 50 and 100 percent of these responses being common to their experience.

It was mentioned earlier about the need to sensitively balance hope with realism; when, where and what to tell the patient about prognosis and diagnosis; achieving a balance between leaving an acceptable level of hope without colluding with false or unjustified expectations of improvement. The inability to accept the reality and permanence of loss of sight has been demonstrated as a key factor in assisting or blocking the overall adjustment pattern of the affected individual. This premise has greater poignancy when it is considered that the highest level of deterioration reported in this category was found in 46 patients, who felt they still longed to be able to see again two years later. It is not possible within the parameters of this book to ascertain the manner in which prognosis may have been explained to this group. It is a natural human response to yearn for what is lost. It would be unhelpful to needlessly go on ceaselessly longing for what can never be. In this study only two people out of 46 felt they were able to cease this longing. Table 6.6 speaks volumes. In virtually every instance there is evidence of deterioration which remained constant over time. It is suggested that such an entrenched pattern of deterioration indicates the need for more counselling and psychological intervention than has previously been considered. Historically, the main thrust of care and rehabilitation has been practical assistance. The evidence of this research, particularly from this material, suggests that a more fruitful allocation of intervention would be focused towards intra-psychic and personal rehabilitation to loss of sight (see Table 6.6)

Self image

Earlier in the chapter we explored possible attributes and circumstances which go to make up or create one's self-image and considered whether one's self-image as a disabled person has any relationship to an individual's former perception of self as an able-bodied person and his or her previously held views about other disabled people. There seemed to be some discrepancy in the sorts of difficulties and degree of affect experienced by those interviewed. For example, 28 patients, over a quarter of the total group, reported feeling embarrassed generally since their loss of sight. Perhaps fortunately, there did not appear to be a direct correlation between this finding and the fact that a much smaller group, 11 patients, felt like a second-class person, of which ten felt no longer socially acceptable. It was noted that there was no improvement in terms of embarrassment or of

Table 6.6. Denial, despair, anger, bitterness, refusal to accept, rejection

Denial, despair, anger, bitterness refusal to accept, rejection	Number out of total group (Base Line 104)	
	Incidence of improvement since loss of sight	Incidence of deterioration since loss of sight and when interviewed
Nothing to get up for	-	17
Nothing to look forward to	3	26
Meaning and purpose had left life	2	23
What had I done to deserve it?	-	31
Why me?	-	33
No hope for the future	3	26
Felt it was unfair	-	31
Thought of taking my life	2	5
Made suicide attempt	1	1
Felt world had crumbled	3	16
Felt no hope for the future	-	20
Someone else to blame	-	11
Bitter about loss of sight	2	24
Felt angry	4	15
Felt sad	3	34
Felt I would not feel again	1	11
Felt nothing worse could happen	-	20
Afraid I would go mad	2	7
Could not cope with anything else.	-	9
Could not accept that it had happened to me	3	35
Could not accept sight would not return	4	26
Felt could have done more to prevent this	-	7
Longing to be able to see	2	46
Would promise to do anything to get my sight back again	-	17

feeling acceptable for any of those in the group when interviewed. It appeared that these responses were directly linked to loss of sight and remained a chronic factor. Society's wider attitudes and stereotypes about disability might begin to explain the basis for such an intractable low self-image and response. Twelve patients experienced severe difficulty with issues of self-image with 28 showing a lesser reaction. Two-fifths of the group experienced minimal problems concerning their identity and self-image; the remainder no answer (see Table 6.7).

Worries about relationships with others

It became apparent that smaller numbers of people were bothered about how their disability would affect their relationships with others. The greatest level of deterioration in 18 patients was fear that others would pity them. Only one lady noted improvement in this respect but felt disinclined to elaborate when requested. The second largest group, fourteen patients, expressed fear that people would reject them. In this group there was no reported incidence of improvement. Perhaps fear of rejection or pity is bound

Table 6.7. Self image

Self image	Number out of total group (Base Line 104)	
	Incidence of improvement since loss of sight	Incidence of deterioration since loss of sight and when interviewed
Felt embarrassed	-	28
Felt ashamed	2	15
Did not like myself	2	6
Felt no longer acceptable	-	10
Felt a second class person	2	11
Felt so alone in this experience	2	28

up with uncertainty about how one should behave towards other people. A frequent concern was how others would perceive them now, following the disability. Fear of pity or rejection may prompt a disabled person, consciously or otherwise, to overcompensate, proving that they can 'go it alone' and are still capable, if not more so, than their sighted peers. Fear of pity might foster an unnecessary prickliness of independence which in turn ironically increases the pressure on the disabled person. Whilst ten people found that they were unsure about what people would expect of them following loss of sight, only two of these reported an improvement, suggesting an increase of confidence over the two year period attributed to intensive rehabilitation. Eight people were uncertain about how to behave with other people, with only one gentleman reporting improvement in his social interactions (see Table 6.8).

Negative changes in social relationships

Just under a third of the group, 33 patients, felt that since loss of sight people expected them to have got used to their disability. Twenty-four commented that since loss of sight and when interviewed, they felt no-one understood what they were going through: only two people suggested an improvement in this respect. This may relate back to our finding that a substantial number of people within the group had difficulty in discussing their worries and

Table 6.8. Worries about relationships with others

Worries about relationships with others	Number out of total group (Base Line 104)	
	Incidence of improvement since loss of sight	Incidence of deterioration since loss of sight and when interviewed
Afraid people would reject me	-	14
Afraid others would pity me	1	18
I tried to cover the fact that I could not see	-	26
I would not be attractive to anyone	-	9
Never to be able to initiate relationships again	-	5
Unsure what people would expect of me	2	10
Did not know how to behave with others	1	8

anxieties with others. Whilst seven reported that family relationships had changed for the worse, it was noted that a further 15 felt that their families did not expect much of them since loss of sight. Some felt people talked down to them and it was apparent that their views had not changed with time. Furthermore, 17 people felt that people generally tried to over-protect them and only one felt this had positively altered over time.

It is clear that these issues are interwoven with those of self-identity and image. What others expect of us or how they perceive and relate to us, will substantially affect our view of our potential and identity within society. When thinking about the seven patients who experienced difficulties with family relationships following loss of sight, perhaps there is a need for intervention allied to personal counselling and practical rehabilitation such as family therapy. (see Table 6.9).

Conclusions

In all seven areas of response as outlined in this chapter, there have been instances of both improvement and deterioration. Sadly, though not surprisingly, deterioration generally outweighs improvement. The most striking features of this chapter demonstrate that by far the greatest difficulty experienced by patients was in relation to inner emotional needs: the ability to come to terms with what has happened, to accept intellectually their loss of

Table 6.9. Negative changes in social relationships

Negative changes in social relationships	Number out of total group (Base Line 104)	
	Incidence of improvement since loss of sight	Incidence of deterioration since loss of sight and when interviewed
People expect me to be used to it.	-	33
People expect me to be grateful	1	12
People would not let me be myself.	1	19
No-one understood what I was going through	2	24
Relationship with family changed for the worse	-	7
People try to overprotect me	1	17
People have no faith in me	-	7
People talk down to me	-	8
Family did not expect much of me	-	15

sight. Consequently, a wide variety of potentially maladaptive responses, some chronic in nature, were evident. The aggregated results from all sections suggests that 79 patients experienced gross deterioration in all sections; only four people appeared to have used the crisis of loss of sight as a positive opportunity and felt that the overall quality of life had improved over time following the initial shock. Small though this latter group is, their ability to make positive use of a critical life event merits further exploration in its own right. Regrettably, it was not possible within the scope of this study to explore such issues as early childhood, rearing and environmental factors in order to understand any possible outcome of loss of sight. The nature and nurture debate still flows on and the essential complexity of man is tantalizingly illusive. A larger study might hopefully one day seek to elucidate such factors.

Recommendations

1. The findings from the holistic assessment suggests that quality of life is markedly affected following loss of sight. The greatest difficulties were experienced in the areas of emotional and intellectual acceptance and adjustment.

2. The study recommends that at both local and national level policy decisions and resource allocation could be appropriately re-evaluated, and that where possible service provision be altered to meet the intra-psychic needs of clients.

3. Whilst practical rehabilitation is obviously important, it is suggested that for too long it had dominated and excluded other aspects of rehabilitation and re-orientation of visually impaired people.

4. The results from this study indicate that clients' needs could be far better met by addressing these subtle, potentially damaging and intractable problems, such as chronic emotional dis-ease and depressive responses to loss of sight.

Chapter 7

Counselling and What It Means

Introduction

Julie Shaw in her study which was primarily concerned with the efficiency and impact of the current registration process upon visually impaired registrants in one southern county in England, comments as follows:

> The system seemed unable to identify clients in urgent need of aid and support, and as a result some benefits came too late; for example, counselling and support during the onset of blindness. Had this been provided earlier, some people would have been helped a lot. (1.1) (Refer also to Chapters 8 and 9 for discussion.)

Furthermore, out of the 86 respondents in her study 7 percent commented that no counselling had been given when they, the clients, thought it was most needed. Similarly, this present study found that of the 104 patients over one-third felt they would have welcomed counselling and emotional help, both at the time of loss and up to two years later when interviewed. This chapter will address these issues by attempting to define 'counselling' and to consider the possible efficiency for visually impaired people and their families. This will encompass discussion about how such a service may best be provided and by whom. The possible structure of a multi- disciplinary counselling service along with patients' perceptions of counselling will be considered. The presentation of case material will elaborate specific coun-selling aims and techniques, and in so doing attempt to clarify what con-stitutes healthy adjustment to visual impairment. The cost effectiveness of counselling will be explored in relation to scarce resource allocation and the implications for local authority social services and regional health auth-orities. The chapter will conclude with recommendations for training and policy decision making.

Before offering various definitions of counselling and discussing its place in the total rehabilitation programme for visually handicapped people and their families, certain themes need clarifying.

It should be stressed that this book is not suggesting that all visually impaired people require counselling—far from it. Two-thirds of the group felt they did not require counselling, which might suggest that for many clients the existing provision is sufficient to meet their needs. Alternatively, it could imply that this group held uncertain or adverse views about counselling. Many individuals will be helped by just one or two sessions for general advice, information giving and the opportunity to off-load. In the earlier sections we have considered the value of crisis intervention, particularly at the point of registration.

This study recognises that a level of informal, well-intentioned befriending with underlying connections with the counselling process, is being offered by specialist workers in the field.

Nor should the impression be conveyed that counselling is the most important component of rehabilitation and re-orientation; all levels of adjustment have equal value and weight in the process of coming to terms with loss of sight. In the case presentations of Mary and Lottie, discussed later, it will be noted that internal psychic adjustment which counselling facilitates can assist the client to make more effective use of practical rehabilitation, being more at ease with self-image, altered social circumstances and the actuality of loss of sight. Counselling, therefore, at whatever level and in whatever form or model used, should really be a forerunner to rehabilitation for daily living. The availability of expert counselling prior to registration is for some clients also crucial for preventive assistance and healthy adjustment, as by the point of registration usually a substantial degree of vision has been lost.

The process of change, including potential loss of employment and independence, may have begun to be confronted with all the attendant stress both for the client and for the family. Arguably then, registration comes too late in the day. For example, a patient with retinitis pigmentosa, whose sight was deteriorating but was not at that time regarded as registerable, requested assistance. The local social services department, although sympathetic, could offer no rehabilitative services unless she was registered. The patient cogently argued that she was feeling exceptionally vulnerable and anxious. In a constructive endeavour she requested both practical rehabilitative services (including braille and mobility skills) and emotional help before her sight deteriorated further. She wanted to prepare herself for the future; to reconstruct her life in order to regain a sense of personal equilibrium. It is important not to make the help provided by social services contingent on the administrative and legislative procedure of registration. Counselling should be consistently available for all visually impaired people who have the motivation and need for it at every stage, both pre- and post-registration.

As will be seen, there are numerous definitions and individual perceptions of what constitutes counselling. The type of counselling intervention may need to vary depending on the client's circumstances. The family also requires help at these times, which might be offered in the form of individual counselling or family/marital therapy, dependent upon the nature of the referral, defined problem and symptoms. One of the main concerns of this project has been to explore clients' needs for emotional support and professional counselling at a time of great crisis, and to gain a sense of how they feel about being on the receiving end of the present system. Arguably there has been in the past a subtle stigma or shame to admit that we, as human beings, might require emotional help in internally adjusting to life crises. Murray-Parkes (1970), Pincus (1976) and others have documented the stiff upper lip tradition in Western cultures in dealing with major loss such as bereavement. Such hesitation and embarrassment in admitting to and owning powerful emotions such as despair, anger and hopelessness, even during prolonged periods of immense upheaval and stress, seem to suggest an in-built fear of showing any natural vulnerability lest we be judged as failures. Whilst such fears are purposely emphasised, nevertheless they are real factors in the context in which counselling operates. Most of us will be familiar with the situation where clients come with a problem, ostensibly of a practical or perceived lesser nature. Through the interview process they are able to bring and share other less tangible difficulties which need ventilating and working through.

The provision therefore of practical rehabilitation services, including mobility training, daily living skills, braille literacy and vocational training—historically the main thrust of care—has colluded with the often unconscious desire to play down the need for help in sustaining emotional equilibrium. Furthermore, counselling *per se* is not a quantifiable activity which can easily be evaluated for either effectiveness or cost efficiency, a point which will be discussed in greater length later. Whilst these issues should be borne in mind, in the last decade particularly the value of interpersonal communication skills and counselling has become increasingly recognised in Western society. This is to be welcomed, but what does counselling mean? There are countless definitions, models and theories, which we may utilise depending on professional background and training or personal experience. Fundamentally the process of counselling has been defined as 'a way of facilitating choice or change or reducing confusion' (1988). At the most simple level counselling is the art of good communication; sensitive, attentive listening with genuinely involved sincere responses. It is two people sharing the same space and time. It is also creating a climate in which clients feel accepted, non-defensive and able to talk freely about themselves and their feelings, and thus begin to build a trusting relationship.

Earlier in the text we have explored the theoretical links between grief following the loss of a loved one (bereavement) and the range of feelings and responses evoked by loss or deterioration of a major sense, such as vision. Before commencing the case discussions of Mary and Lottie, consideration needs to be given to what might be meant by 'healthy, psychological, emotional and intellectual adjustment to loss of sight' by exploring the views of patients in this study.

In attempting to simplify the concept of counselling patients were asked:

Given that loss of vision affects one's overall situation, would it have helped to talk to a skilled person about your feelings and the changes that loss of sight has imposed on you and your family, and to explore new ways of coping? (Interview questionnaire)

Over a third of the 104 patients said they would have welcomed this support. This came as no real surprise given that when we had earlier posed the question 'How do you see the future?' (following registration), the range of responses could be interpreted as being indicative of emotional distress, as well as reflecting their practical circumstances.

One lady, registered as degeneratively blind, said she felt that she was on 'a downward road'. Several replies reverted to the stoical response, implying they had no choice but to grin and bear it. Many said they tried not to think of the future or to plan ahead, living from day to day. This inability to think ahead is a common feature with the bereaved or grieving. It is as though all resources are focused on coping with the here and now. This tendency may be prolonged over months or years.

Other replies reflected a greater sense of despair and uncertainty, ranging from 'I cry all the time' (male, blind), and 'Very bad, no good living, is it?' (female, blind), to 'I can't keep fighting' (female, partially sighted). This lady felt it had been one long battle to get any professional input and practical rehabilitation. She presumably felt unequal to the prospect of requesting counselling. The ambiguity of her reply could also encompass a real sense of her frustration, recorded by the interviewer, that her illness had in some sense emotionally defeated her and she did not feel able to resume the fight for greater independence. Whatever the possibilities, much of this type of investigation has to remain necessarily in the shadowy realms of speculation.

The poignancy of these comments and the isolation they hint at, linked to the third who were clearly stating two years after registration that they would welcome professional counselling, should not pass without comment. Little comfort should be taken from the rest of the group who did not feel they required counselling, as it was found there was some contradictions between what clients had earlier said in the interview and their affirmation that they would not welcome counselling. For example, one partially sighted woman who had repeatedly said the help she most needed was someone to talk with about her feelings about visual impairment, asserted that she had adjusted very well and did not want counselling. It could be assumed she meant she had adjusted well on a practical level. In retrospect this question was too vaguely defined and should have sought to differentiate whether patients had adjusted well practically and/or emotionally.

It is perhaps not surprising that people are unclear about what is meant by counselling, and may confuse this in their minds with social befriending which has links, however tenuous, with the art of counselling. Counselling, which at its core aims to be a warm, empathetic interpersonal communica-

tion, is much more. Counselling is concerned with the purposeful exploration and resolution of internal emotional or psychological distress, ambivalence and conflict, aiming to alleviate potentially maladaptive social and
personal functioning, whilst simultaneously assisting the client to a deeper
level of self awareness, insight and personal potential, thus aiming to
diminish the risk of psychiatric/emotional instability, anguish, or pathological reaction to the loss of sight.

Counselling

The case presentation of Mary [1]

In discussing the practical options open to carers about whether or not, and
to what extent, to provide counselling, presuming adequate counselling
training and supervision are available, let us consider the aims of such
intervention. If the overall aim is defined as 'to promote a healthy psychological, emotional and intellectual adjustment to loss of sight for clients', the
question remains: what is meant by this? The cases of Mary and Lottie might
go some way to clarify this. Mary was a participant in the project, referred
following the initial interview. This 33 year-old West Indian lady had been
registered totally blind some 18 months previously, following acute glaucoma. She had retained residual perception of light and dark. During the
assessment interview Mary informed the interviewer that she felt she had
been blind for three years, despite registration only 18 months previously.
She admitted having avoided any rehabilitation/mobility training as this
reinforced the sense of permanency about her loss of sight. At this time Mary
was adamant that she hoped her sight would return, and felt that the
ophthalmologist had left her with this hope. General understanding was that
this was extremely unlikely. Intellectually, because Mary hoped her sight
would return, she felt no overriding motivation to co-operate with rehabilitation orientation training. On two previous occasions during the last 18
months she had started, then withdrawn from, a mobility training programme. Her experienced and committed technical officer for the blind felt
at a loss how to approach immobilization. At this time Mary expressed a
range of emotions, and abhorrence of meeting other disabled people. She
lived with her elder sister who was her only source of social contact, being
unable to get out alone Mary made her a virtual prisoner in her own flat.
One was forcibly struck by Mary's wit and courage in the face of chronic
depression, isolation and loss of self-esteem and identity. At the close of the
first session it was agreed that she seemed blocked, unable to mourn what
she had lost, or move forward. At this time, Mary described herself as 'dark
and numb inside'. An initial contract was agreed of 12 weekly or fortnightly

---

[1] The counselling model underlying this case presentation is derived from that of
the London Hospital Bereavement Service, though adapted by the author with
reference to disability and loss of sight.

sessions of one hour. The practical focus of intervention had thus far been ineffective because Mary had been unable to feel any level of real acceptance of loss of sight. Depression and low self-esteem had militated against the persistent motivation necessary for healthy resolution and rehabilitation.

During the next four sessions certain aspects of her personality and behaviour were explored. Although intellectually Mary appeared to have accepted the reality of her loss of sight, emotionally she felt disbelief and rage about her handicap. She felt an inability to communicate her feelings of bitterness and resentment about this to others. Because she was increasingly fearful about the intensity of her reactions which had for so long been bottled up she had become a model person according to her internal expectations, outwardly cheerful and full of fun at all times. This, she decided, made others feel better but it involved her biting back the resentment and frustration she so often felt. Giving Mary the opportunity and permission to grieve and acknowledge her own depression, and encouraging her to ventilate her pent up emotions was central to the process of the work. Demonstrating through the counselling relationship that others could withstand her anger and distress, Mary began gradually to tolerate her own reactions to her loss. She began to see her emotions less as a potentially destructive and dangerous force, and more as a natural and healthy, though at times painful, response to the enormous changes in her life.

Mary's intellectual acceptance of her blindness was only superficial. It was apparent from the assessment session that she had continually avoided any action or reference which emphasised her loss of sight. This was tackled by indirect intervention. A health programme was evolved to combat her disrupted sleep pattern and lethargy, incorporating a regime of relaxation exercises, a structured daily routine and the prescribed task to go out on weekly visits to places of local interest with an escort and taking her white stick. This task had several functions which addressed the difficulty of intellectual acceptance. Mary explored her fantasies about emotional public perception of blind people, and the double bind in which she was caught: on the one hand wanting to hide and deny her blindness, and on the other, because of this, being unable to use the rehabilitation training, so essentially become more dependent, isolated and stereotypically blind. We linked her concern with her cultural expectations and perceptions of disability. The role and impact that her family had in early childhood and at the time of her loss of sight was explored and worked through. Mary's intellectual denial appeared in her choice of potential employment—to work in a clothing factory sorting out coloured garments. (Denial can be either an unconscious process or a conscious defence against psychic pain.) By reflecting on her internal feelings of emptiness and darkness in connection with this response she was able, with help, to begin to get in touch with the implicit paradox and denial in wanting to seek employment which would focus on light, sight and colours. Simultaneously, she sought to explore the basis of her self-identity. Since her blindness she had become increasingly aware of always having to measure her achievements in specific time limits. This response is not uncommon; following the onset of any major disability there is a loss of self-confidence and esteem as the disabled person strives to establish a new internal perception of him/herself. This new self-image is constantly shifting in interactional response to the expectations, stereotypes and needs of others around the disabled person. The very real change in social, work and financial status following loss of vision impinges on the new role the disabled person assumes. Any exploration of Mary's identity involved not only her own perceptions but her role within the family and wider society and their response to her. She described herself as someone who was viewed by others as being mentally retarded. She had certainly become a very passive tenant within her own home and resented this, but felt unable to break out of this pattern. By working at Mary's own pace several goals she could strive for were identified:

(a) to become more involved in local voluntary and/or disabled groups as she felt appropriate; and

(b) to redecorate her own bedroom, perhaps using tactile mediums. The covert intention of this goal was to subtly and gently reinforce Mary's new position of visual impairment, whilst reinforcing her active self-determination in these activities with the wider implications for confidence building.

At this time, Mary had begun on the mutually agreed task that she go on weekly trips with an escort and, when feeling comfortable, taking her white stick—not to use as a mobility aid but to explore her feelings about it—and to try to consider what new pleasures/elements she got out of these trips using other senses. To her amazement she found that in spite of her disability she was able to contribute to and gain a lot from these activities. The counsellor could see that Mary's depression was lifting and she was becoming more assertive and confident of her right to express herself and to determine her future.

Characteristically, Mary displayed a need to play down her achievements and obvious progress, which is not an uncommon response for people moving out of grief and depression following a major loss or change. This denial of improvement or progress can be attributed to what has been described in analytical terms as resistance to change. Change in itself can be potentially threatening, even if the established emotional response and behaviour is viewed as a problem. For example, although she had the insight to accept that her isolation, depression and sense of worthlessness was counter-productive as well as extremely painful, it was at least familiar, something adopted following the crisis of sight loss. One of her worries centred around what would replace the depression. Furthermore, when struggling to work through depression there can be an attendant fear of failure of not being able to change. Therefore a perverse logic may unconsciously operate—'if I never try to change then I can't be said to fail the attempt'. At such times this underlying anxiety and resistance to change must be acknowledged and therapeutically contained.

By the sixth session Mary was taking her white stick out whenever she left the flat and she was becoming increasingly involved with a local Physically Handicapped and Able Bodied (PHAB) group; she had been asked to sit on the organising committee, an obvious boost to her self-confidence. A significant shift at this time was that Mary, unknown to the counsellor or rehabilitation worker, attended an interview for a training course unescorted. This obvious achievement highlighted Mary's repairing confidence, and the determination and tenacity she had to cope with these two potentially challenging situations. The pleasure and self-perpetuating reinforcement she experienced in recounting these triumphs were obvious and perhaps 'curative'. These qualities supported the counsellor's earlier conviction on first meeting Mary, namely that she possessed depths of determination and resilience which only needed reactivating to show the true potential of this courageous and likable woman.

An important facet of any counselling alliance is to gain the subtle balance between positively reinforcing improvement and effort in exploring very painful issues, while gently reaffirming the client's need/right to fluctuate emotionally in relation to past crises and the current changes taking place.

Therefore, working through grief, which includes internalizing and making sense of traumatic life events, can be likened to the flow and ebbs of tides: never ending but with each constant flow from day to day affecting the change. The role of counselling can help to direct that flow, allowing clients to achieve the change in their own unique way. In this way clients decide for themselves what is a feasible and comfortable level of tolerance, as opposed to passive acceptance, in coping with loss of vision, and in so doing move forward to new possibilities.

The last three sessions in Mary's case were used to review:

(a) where she had metaphorically come from since commencing counselling, and

(b) where she wanted to go: 'what the future held for her'.

The explored her role and responsibility in shaping her future, tempered with a realistic appraisal of what rehabilitation services, employment options and social situations awaited her. By the eighth session Mary had commenced mobility training and was working intensively with her technical officer, liaising with agencies in a programme of practical rehabilitation.

At the close of the ninth session Mary was significantly independent in caring for herself: mobile and independent in her local area and increasingly involved in community activities for both the able bodied and disabled groups. At review, three months later, she had a place on a commercial training course and eventually gained a job in the voluntary sector.

This account is not intended to constitute a glib success story about counselling. The fact that Mary got from Point A to Point B with much heartache and hard work on her part along the way says much about her as a person. She entered fully into the counselling contract in every sense of the word. However, if we conclude this account with an appraisal of progress made, we begin to see what may constitute a healthier all-round adjustment to loss of sight. The major themes will be constant with the fine details changing from person to person and situation to situation, dependent upon the counselling model used, the theoretical perspective, experience and training of counsellors involved and, most importantly, dependent upon the clients themselves and their motivation to make use of counselling and the experiences from which they come.

At the end of the counselling intervention Mary had begun to grasp and tolerate the long term implications of her disability and, equally important, to tentatively explore her own internal emotional responses. The newfound insight presented Mary with a choice—to allow herself to be more comfortable with her more infantile needs and to accept that a level of dependency can be a cathartic experience. At the conclusion of counselling Mary felt that she wanted to explore the possibility of long term psychotherapy to address more deeply rooted unresolved issues from her past which had affected her response to disability. Counselling, it appeared, had given her a sense of direction (see Table 7.1).

The case presentation of Lottie [2]

Lottie was referred by the consultant physician treating her for diabetes. In his opinion this 39 year-old Asian lady was struggling to maintain her condition. It was felt that this was a consequence of her ambivalence and extreme distress about her diabetes and rapidly deteriorating vision, and combined with these difficulties were marital problems. Lottie was an attractive, garrulous and vivacious lady. There was always a prevailing sense, however, that this bright exterior was illusive and brittle. She was both enthusiastic and committed to the idea of counselling, and in the first sessions was able to share her past circumstances and her concerns. She had emigrated to this country at the age of 21 in order to continue her studies in English literature. Soon after she had met and married a fellow Asian student who had subsequently trained and qualified as a care worker. At the time counselling commenced she had been married for some 12 years.

Prior to developing diabetes some three years earlier, Lottie had received the devastating news that she was infertile. The couple had been desperately trying for a family for some years and their mounting suspicions had led them to seek specialist help. In Lottie's cultural terms this, she felt, rendered

[2] The identifying details of the counsellee, here called 'Lottie', have been altered for confidentiality. Any resemblance to person or persons is coincidental and not intended. These case presentations are offered for training purposes only.

Table 7.1. Assessment overview

Dimension	Prior to counselling	Counselling intervention	Outcome
Emotional	Unable to express anger/feelings = depression etc.	Encourage to ventilate/mourn loss. Test that others can withstand her distress not destructive.	Able to share feelings with others, tolerate own response, increased self-assertion.
Intellectual	Superficial acceptance of loss and permanency = defence against pain and grief denial.	Explored internal darkness/upheaval with external reality —worked through.	Began to tolerate reality and permanence of loss, accepted rehabilitation/ mobility training.
Identity	Damaged self-image, loss of self-self-confidence/ esteem.Perceived self as worth less or retarded.	1) Client defined skills/attributes. 2) explored social networkconfidence. 3) structured daily routine 4) client defined possibilities for increased social contact.	Client self-motivated gained interview/ training/employment, increased self-confidence. Expanded social network.
Philosophical	No previous strong faith, felt mistrustful of life.	Considered implications for 1, 2 and 3 above.	Client evolved a more questioning outlook and philosophy of life reappraising questions about injustice/fate etc.
Family Network	Unable to be 'self', very passive but resentful.	Worked through via open/closed question and increased sight into family's needs etc., and role play, 1 and 2 above.	Less family tension. Mary more open and assertive. Four months after contract, Mary rehoused on her own.
Health	1) Disrupted sleep pattern. 2) Lethargic. 3) Poor appetite = anxiety, depression.	5) Relaxation exercise program. 6) Daily exercise. 7) Structured routine (links to 2 and 3).	Gained physical equilibrium. Sleep stabilized. Planning for the future.
Practical Rehabilitation	Refused mobility training/practical rehabilitation/ orientation training. 'Prisoner in my own home.'	Integrated above (1 concepts to 7). Client liaised with Technical Officer.	1) Independent mobility. 2) Gained employment. 3) Self-determining

her useless as a woman, barren and unproductive as a wife. It seemed that she and her husband had not been able to allow themselves to properly take in or come to terms with this first disclosure before the initial onset of diabetes made itself felt. With the decline in her health Lottie's sense of worthlessness deepened. It was with a more real sense of sadness that she allowed herself slowly to disclose and own her feelings of loss and emptiness. Her husband began to work long periods away from home, a fact which Lottie accepted with resignation, feeling it was his right as she had failed him. It was passively accepted that their marriage was under great strain and that her husband was considering separation. Lottie's perception was that he blamed her both for her infertility and for the diabetes. The mounting tension of these unspoken accusations was steadily but systematically undermining their ability to communicate. It appeared there was persistent mutual collusion about not working on their marital/sexual problems as both felt it to be pointless and refused marital therapy.

It appeared also that Lottie colluded with her husband's perception of her as a failure, and she accepted that it was his cultural right to seek a more fertile wife with whom he could produce a family. At a deeper level there was a sense in which Lottie would not allow herself to grieve over these traumatic events, or to acknowledge the pain that the breakup in their relationship might potentially cause.

Although the initial counselling referral had been precipitated by concern over maintenance of her diabetes, it was clear that these factors were the tip of an iceberg and could not be explored in isolation to the other major losses in her life. At the commencement of counselling Lottie, though academically well-qualified, had found it extremely difficult to find suitable employment. She was reading with the utmost difficulty despite the support of low visual aids. Living primarily on her own, mobility had become a greater problem for which she had sought training. These increasing practical incapacitations, linked to her home and social circumstances, all militated towards undermining Lottie's diminishing confidence.

Counselling was commenced on an open-ended weekly basis with initial agreement that Lottie needed to allow some space to reflect on other long term losses which might be fuelling her inability to care for herself and colour her attitude towards diminished vision. There was speculation that her lack of self-care maintenance was an unconscious depressive response indicating unexpressed self-destructive urges, or suicidal tendency. This was explored early on, though initially denied by Lottie, and rationalized as her forgetfulness to take medication. It was important to hear and respect her rationalization as a possible defense.

Lottie's early childhood had been spent on a farm in India. The youngest of six children, she viewed her childhood as settled and happy despite her family existing on scarce resources. What emerged gradually but increasingly was a picture of a child who had existed on scarce resources in more ways than one. Being the youngest, the elder siblings were assigned to look after her. Although physical care was adequate there was a sense in which warmth and personal intimacy on a day to day basis was often lacking due to the many pressures which waylaid the family. Being a bright child she had won a scholarship and had become the unexpected vehicle for the family ambition to receive an education in England. Their pride in her appeared to fit and fuel her need for approval and her longing for adventure. This honour was double- edged for Lottie. On the one hand for the first time she felt singled out as special, and on the other she felt an enormous pressure to achieve and live up to family expectations and dreams.

The disclosure of her infertility and knowledge of her progressive physical condition had, Lottie felt, essentially blocked her ability to fulfil not only her dreams but those of her family. Lottie felt she had failed herself, her husband and her family—a heavy burden to carry. What came across was the feeling that she existed only in terms of other's approval of her, and any sense of self-worth she gained came from the praise and acknowledgement of others not an easily innate quality, though perhaps sadly surprising given her background.

A life tapestry of multiple disappointment and loss began to show itself. Time and life's circumstance had never allowed for working through her feelings about her childhood and relationships to her parents. The leaving of her homeland and her culture was something that had barely been acknowledged. It had been defended against by being perceived only in terms of a positive adventure. The diagnosis of infertility and diabetes had seemingly served to reinforce Lottie's view that she was 'rotten' at the core. This self-description might be translated into her lost sense of femininity. Equally, it could be suggestive of an unconscious acknowledgement of psychic vulnerability or damage. Both possibilities were silently noted by the counsellor and held until such times as Lottie was able to use and tolerate such suggestions. There was also a prevailing feeling from Lottie that having been was given a disability was God's judgement. Though acknowledged as irrational, this preoccupation was forceful and pervasive. Lottie was keen to assert that she bore no ill-will or sense of injustice or anger either towards her husband for his response or to any other protagonist in her life's circumstances. There was a sense in which resignation of fate masked powerful feelings.

One of the aims of counselling was to offer her an alternative perspective of her behaviour and the inherent contradictions which appeared to be around. It appeared that Lottie would split off and deny both negative feelings and concordant behaviour. For example, whilst overtly appearing very resigned to her fate, on one level denying anxiety and presenting herself as quite meek and mild, in essence she was a very powerful lady in engaging numerous agencies to offer support. It appeared that she had a way of provoking intense anxiety and pity and was quite vocal in demanding her rights as she perceived them from various statutory and voluntary organisations offering support. The apparent split between her overt behaviour and conscious perceptions of herself, and the behaviour she engaged in may have served to illustrate this as a way of splitting and off-loading (projecting) anger and frustration onto other extraneous forces. Lottie was continually dogged by irritation at what she saw as ineffective and insufficient service provision. At times these paranoiac sounding perceptions delighted in frustrating her demands. Such feelings might serve as a visible window into the real depths of her inner child, frustration, despair and rage. The counsellor speculated and wondered why such frustrations appeared to be reserved for other professionals/agencies. What was the essence and purpose of this? What might it demonstrate about her feelings in session? Why was there a need to have a split between the resigned, meek image and the demanding political reformer. Such work was necessarily very slow, and at times arduous for both Lottie and the counsellor. This might have been Lottie's way of conveying to the counsellor that she did not feel sufficiently held or emotionally contained in session. This needy lady's anxiety was being acted out in trying to gain access to several sources of perceived help. It was as if she was saying 'I am afraid that one counsellor is not going to be enough to cope with all the pain and terror I feel, so I had better share it around'. It was a very long time before Lottie was ready to hear this, and even longer before she was able to retrospectively admit the possibility of it.

In such instances it is important for the counsellor to keep listening with an inner ear, both to what is not being spoken by the patient—attempting to grasp unconscious messages that might be abroad—and to the feelings that are alive in the here and now. What feelings are aroused in the counsellor? What might this tell us about how the patient is feeling at any given time? In working with Lottie, the counsellor frequently had to struggle internally against an overwhelming sense of despair and depression that everything was so hopeless for Lottie that nothing much could be achieved. This had to be understood in terms of projective identification. Simply put, this is a defense mechanism by which the patient manages to unconsciously project into the therapist what it is like to be literally 'in the patient's shoes'. The therapist/counsellor is then able to 'understand' through this intrusive mechanism something of what the patient might be going through at any given stage. It is one of the aims of a therapeutic relationship that anxieties should be acknowledged and held by the therapist's understanding and acceptance of them. When this is inadvertently missed altogether or ill-timed, we might wonder about the counsellor's personal 'baggage' unconsciously intruding in the session, or alternatively that the patient manages to induce the blockage in the counsellor as a way of avoiding what really needs to be verbalized and explored. It might be said that there is always the possibility of a push-pull factor in therapy, with the patient simultaneously wanting, yet resisting, the therapeutic process.

Gradually, as trust steadily deepened between Lottie and the counsellor, it appeared that some of anger was being played out in session. At times she berated the counsellor as useless and incompetent because she felt the counsellor wasn't doing anything practical to help her. Co-existing with these feelings, Lottie also displayed insights about the importance of her having someone to talk through her many confusing feelings.

Lottie's technical officer expressed concern and bewilderment about her apparent inability to present positively at interview. At such times it seemed she became inarticulate tongue-tied and, despite her academic qualifications, could not seem to perform to her intellectual ability. Lottie was able to bring these external concerns and much time was spent exploring the basis of her anxiety. Lottie felt she was trapped in a self-fulfilling circle; she saw herself as a failure and therefore lived up to her own internal critical expectations. To counteract this, the counsellor arranged for a colleague to set up several video sessions to practice interview technique using role play. The boundaries for this were firmly set in that Lottie's task, with her agreement, was to practice being interviewed for imaginary jobs. Her response and feelings in carrying out this task was to be explored within the framework of counselling. Initially, Lottie appeared quite excited by the prospect of being video-taped. The counsellor felt there might be some anxiety underlying this heightened response. The experience of being videoed and watching herself on television proved painful but fruitful. It seemed that Lottie was able for the first time to make a connection between how she saw herself in her fantasy internal imagination and to what was perceived externally. In fantasy Lottie held onto the view of herself as a charismatic, dynamic and forceful person who would bowl over the interviewers naturally, thus requiring little effort on her part to sell herself. Conversely, a much more negative fantasy of herself was clearly operating; that it was pointless trying to present herself in a good light as she was a pathetic object of pity that other people would perceive as a 'dummy'. Through many painful and harrowing sessions Lottie was able to explore with the counsellor the reality of how she presented on video film. The counsellor strove to highlight positive qualities whilst gently challenging Lottie's more punitive and negative view of herself. In this way, the aim was to both bolster ego strength and to reinforce a more positive self-image. In all Lottie undertook three sessions of role play which were then linked into the counselling programme.

Much of the work was to assist Lottie to mourn her many losses. It is important to be realistic about what therapy or counselling can achieve in the face of so much pain and long term accumulative distress. Lottie's response to her diabetes and deteriorating eyesight was bound up with mourning the loss of her homeland, coming to terms with the sadness about lack of family love, awareness of her infertility and marital breakup. Counselling sought to help Lottie hold onto an equilibrium, forestalling mental breakdown. The fact that Lottie was continuing to function at all, and more importantly by the end of counselling containing her diabetes, was realistically an achievement for her and perhaps the most she could manage at that time. Lottie's sight would continue to deteriorate and her emotional response would vary in accordance. Anxiety was displayed from time to time by Lottie contacting multiple agencies in an attempt to engage support when she felt particularly vulnerable or fearful of being out of control. She chose to discontinue counselling, which was respected by the counsellor, as Lottie felt she was managing to cope. At one level it could be that her desire to cease counselling was in fact a flight into health: a fear of becoming too dependent on the counsellor. Whilst acknowledging this possibility to Lottie, the counsellor felt it was also important to hear her need to authorise autonomy and control over the situation. She had begun the work of understanding herself and coming to terms with very difficult life circumstances. However, there was much more that might have been achieved and it was hoped that in the future Lottie would decide to return to counselling as and when she felt it necessary.

Earlier in this chapter brief mention was made of counselling and cost efficiency, which is complicated by many factors. The present economic and social climate calling for bureaucratic and administrative prudence and accountability has had visible repercussions on service provision in local government. Local authority social service departments and welfare agencies have not been immune; consequently during the last decade they have been compelled to rationalize their service. Furthermore, growing public awareness of and concern about the statutory responsibilities of social work practice (child care and mental health) which have been reflected in media coverage of tragic fatalities, have placed even greater pressures on local authorities, social service management and social workers to ensure that these areas of work are given paramount priority. This picture is further complicated by difficulty in recruiting entrants to social work training and practice in some urban areas and the growing reported trend of experienced workers either leaving the profession or migrating away from urban areas. These factors may be said to set the scene when rationalizing scarce resources of finance and staff. It is acknowledged that more than ever before social workers and other carers have to be seen to get results. It is from this context that evaluation of counselling and its cost efficiency have to be considered. The case against counselling in such a climate could be put, with some justification, as follows:

1. Counselling is a costly resource in terms of training, supervision and especially in the time expended on individual clients.

2. The nature of the task of counselling does not easily lend itself to objective evaluation.

3. The benefits of counselling are hidden, i.e. known uniquely to the counselled individual. There is no quantifiable evidence to submit for scrutiny when vying for the allocation of scarce resources.

4. If the benefits of counselling are hidden, then by implication the need for such help is subjective; i.e. people may survive without counsell-

ing. Surviving with distress or with maladaptive behaviour rather than achieving an adequate quality of life.

5. Current facilities are utilized fully and are hard put to meet existing demands.

What are the merits of these arguments in relation to services for the visually impaired?

The first, second and fifth points are central to the provision of counselling for any client group. If, however, the cost can be offset against savings in other areas by the effective and purposeful use of other facilities, then the cost looks more attractive. Let us consider this in relation to Mary's situation prior to the instigation of counselling. Mary had been visited regularly by various rehabilitation workers from social services; she had resisted all their efforts to motivate her and said she gained little from the costly residential rehabilitation centre she attended. The aids and adaptions provided had been largely unused. She had resisted learning braille as she had previously said that braille dots felt like 'pins in her fingers'—another symptom of Mary's internal distress and conflict with external reality. These resources were not used appropriately or effectively prior to counselling. Fitzgerald in an earlier study (1970) links unhealthy adjustment to inability to use the aids provided; for example, 33 out of his 66 respondents had not used the white sticks provided. Thurme and Murphree (1961) found that acceptance of a white stick was a predictor of healthy adjustment to loss of sight. There has been documentation citing some local authorities who despatch white sticks through the post, ostensibly to reduce spending. Such misinformed manoeuvres are fated to be ineffective and wasteful. Furthermore, this is setting aside the personal impact on the newly registered visually impaired population who are treated in this way.

Related research on emotional responses to physical handicap shows a similar trend. A strikingly high percentage of artificial prostheses supplied, particularly for the upper body, remain wrapped and unused. One can speculate about the similarities and underlying cause for such behaviour.

Even though existing services may be utilized fully, this is not the same as their being utilized to the best effect. Counselling may be able to facilitate the more purposeful use of aids and other rehabilitative services.

Finally, what should determine how resources are allocated? Society's expectations or individual need as defined by the users? Such consideration calls for a more detailed debate about the reliability of consumers' and workers' perceptions of need and the most appropriate intervention.

Sainsbury's comment has resonance with the above issues:

> In the face of the complexity of social and political analysis one can at least assert that what happens to people as individuals should be a matter of concern and interest; that, in assessing what is good one should not wholly be guided by the numbers of people directly or indirectly affected; and—as a corollary of this—that a public opinion

poll is not a sufficient guide of itself to what should or should not be done in public service terms nor to the evaluation of service activities. (1983)

It is the author's belief that ultimately the effectiveness of counselling for the visually impaired, as for any other group, can only truly be assessed in terms of individual (micro) benefit. However, the commitment to and formation of policies on a macro level to instigate counselling as a precursor to rehabilitation would allow, at least, the opportunity for systematic examination of its potential.

Who should provide a counselling service

The question of who is best placed to provide counselling for the visually impaired has to be explored in the knowledge of all those professional and voluntary workers who come into contact with this group. Traditionally there has been the assumption on the part of specialist rehabilitation workers that counselling is an unofficial aspect of their role. However, until very recently very little, if any, specific counselling training was integrated in the training course. The impression prevailing was of somewhat woolly thinking surrounding the differences between befriending, supporting, talking and counselling. Whilst the first three may be rightly said to be components of the latter, there are distinct differences as previously discussed.

Is it an appropriate role for rehabilitation or mobility officers employed by the local authority social services whose focus is arguably a deterministic, educative role—imparting new skills and adaptive solutions to practical issues of daily concerns? The author wonders whether combining this role with counselling may be expecting too much of these workers. Is there a conflict of roles between non-directive counselling, where the client is encouraged to be self-determining and explorative, and the over didactic role of rehabilitation workers who offer training? Can they wear both hats comfortably? What effect might this have on the counselling contract where the client has to cope with relating to the same worker in different roles? These questions have yet to be systematically and empirically explored, but should be borne in mind when considering the complex question of liaison between specialist workers, generic social workers and the concerns of medical and nursing personnel. One possible solution, which will be elaborated further in the next section, is to offer a multi- disciplinary counselling training programme where all professionals involved in the care of the visually handicapped can expand their existing knowledge and skills in counselling, having cumulative beneficial impact on patients as they progress through the system. Clients could be referred to a cohesively structured counselling and rehabilitative service.

Such a service would need to ensure both confidentiality and anonymity in some of its aspects. The trained counsellor could be a technical officer, ophthalmic nurse, social worker or general practitioner, whose particular professional experience would be complemented in training by appreciation of the implications of loss of sight for the individual and family. Importantly, the allocated counsellor who would be 'matched' to the client would not automatically be the client's key professional worker. With the client's consent and knowledge, liaison between all professionals would be encouraged as appropriate. Such a system would provide the client/family with an opportunity to explore and ventilate any particular issues or difficulties encountered in contacts with other professionals. In this way the counsellor may facilitate preventative adaptive responses, identifying with the client what is best to be done in the circumstances.

In helping carers to meet the various and complex needs of this group, there is a need to impart a range of special skills which can be learnt and which involve specific assessment and counselling techniques. Such training could also be provided through post qualification study. Assessing prospective counsellors' motivation, personal needs, skills and past life-experience when applying for counselling training is most vital, as well as encouraging them to experience counselling and therapy for themselves in order to work through unresolved issues. The curriculum should provide both a general and theoretical understanding of loss/change counselling models, how to achieve a changed response to crisis, and an intensive practical experience of assessment techniques and interviewing skills. Such training should impart a minimum standard of proficiency in counselling skills, followed by an integrated assessment and probationary period. Most important, there should be on-going supervision of counsellors' practice. This provides the support they need, enhancing professional development in skills and experience.

Conclusions and recommendations

1. Rehabilitative assistance and counselling (where provided) offered by social service departments should not be contingent on the client being registered or suitable for registration as visually impaired.
2. Access to specialist services should be available both before and after registration.
3. Counselling should be an available precursor to rehabilitation, thereby potentially increasing the likelihood of effective practical intervention.
4. Post qualification specific and general study in counselling techniques should be more widely available, possibly on the basis of in-service training.
5. The collaboration of all professionals involved in the care of the visually impaired would have healthy beneficial ripple effects for the client group as they move through the system.

6. The instigation of a structured multi-disciplinary counselling service would provide cross fertilization of experience, making paragraph 3 above more a reality than an ideal.[3]

7. The philosophy underlying resource allocation should be enriched by concern with meeting 'internal' needs and concerns, with the emphasis shifting away from mainly quantifiable, 'external' and visible provision and activity.

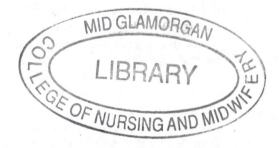

[3] The suggested model for a multi-disciplinary counselling service is drawn from the London Hospital Voluntary Bereavement Counselling Service.

Chapter 8

New Roads Lie Ahead
Rehabilitative After Care Services

Introduction

Brief consideration has been given to the part played by social services in processing registration papers, Form BD8. It was encouraging to note that 39 people had been visited prior to registration which is undoubtedly good preventative practice. Such early intervention allows for a thorough assessment and long term planning with the client about a range of services and support they and their families might require in the future. It has been considered in previous chapters that deteriorating vision can undermine an individual's confidence, self-identity and sense of personal value. In the last chapter a specific model of counselling which addresses such responses was considered in order to highlight the contribution that carers can make when utilising counselling skills. It is, however, important to stress here that early assessment may provide a frame of reference for both clients and their families about what services are available, what training is possible and, where appropriate, identifying what vocational rehabilitation might be called for; these combined reflections may considerably strengthen the affected individual's sense of self-esteem, allowing him or her to be vocal and self-determining in making short, medium and long term decisions and choices. It is important not to underestimate the contribution that social workers and other professionals can make at this early stage. Penelope Shaw (1985) has rightly commented that many clients will not necessarily have access to specialist social work support and that generic social workers generally may only have a hazy understanding of the social implications and potentialities for their clients who are facing loss of sight. In her study of the registration process in one southern county in England Julie Shaw noted that just under half the respondents in her survey felt there had been lack of information from social services. Those individuals also criticised their social workers' lack of knowledge of specific eye conditions, of the registration process itself and what benefits and services they would be entitled to as a consequence of registration. Such observations linked to the findings of this study, which will be discussed later in this chapter, may well have implications for social work training; they certainly imply the need for generic social workers to be given an induction in-service training on specific aspects of disability which includes a basic understanding of the implications of visual impairment, registration and rehabilitation.

Evaluating clients' perceptions of the rehabilitation services provided by social services departments necessarily gives rise to constructive criticism, nevertheless retaining an awareness of the context in which such assistance is offered. Bearing in mind restricted resources, the prevailing staff-client ratio, the general bombardment rate of referrals and, most particularly, the statutory demands placed upon departments in relation to mental welfare, family and child abuse work, such limitations force pressurised management and front line workers to continually review, evaluate and prioritize their provisions and intervention. In such a climate it seems sadly inevitable that decisions will be made daily about which client group is most in need of intensive or specialised assistance. There are no easy choices to be made in such circumstances. This study set out to explore the untested assumption that social work support for visually handicapped people, as part of the larger physically disabled client group, is seen as a poor relation in main stream welfare practice. Given that in Julie Shaw's study and in this study also, only a small minority saw any advantage in registration, it therefore seemed necessary to investigate the main causes for the apparent ineffectiveness of this process. The need to review the services which registration offers access to seemed relevant.

In attempting to assess the continuum of care offered by social services departments, clients were asked how they coped before assistance was offered. The aim was to define how patients and their families managed on a day to day basis in the interim period following the registration examination at the hospital.

Clients' perceptions of the type of help and assistance they felt they needed, and the sort of care they were actually offered and eventually received is compared and contrasted. Clients' reflections about who most helped them work through their feelings and difficulties about loss of sight will be set alongside these other lines of investigation. The chapter will conclude with an assessment of how clients viewed the future after rehabilitation and in so doing seek to identify common themes of improvement, quality of life and difficulty in psychological and social adjustment to disability.

Ultimately, the predominant aim and focus of this chapter is to explore to what extent social work intervention met clients' broader psychological and emotional needs. Donnelly (1986), Penelope Shaw (1985) and others have extensively reviewed rehabilitation services within Great Britain. As mentioned in the foreword of this work, little emphasis has been placed hitherto on systematically investigating intra-personal needs and responses following loss of sight. As such, whilst the full range of services offered to clients will be discussed, and is given credence as being crucial to overall healthy resolution of the changes, it is not the central and overriding aim of this study to re-state much of what has been documented elsewhere about daily living skills etc.

Clients' perceptions of how they managed before assistance was provided

The commonest response from the clients concerning how they managed in the interim period between registration at the hospital and awaiting first contact from social services department, was one of stoicism. Nearly two-thirds of the total group had to wait for several weeks for a visit from their social services department. Many clients spoke of muddling through in the best way they could, or commented that friends and families had given them a lot of support at this time. For some, the realistic response was that registration had not qualitatively changed their life in any way as their visual deterioration was spread over many months or years. Some spoke with pride of their achievements in coping during this period:

> 'I used to find it difficult, but I tried to do it myself. I managed a bit.'

> 'I managed okay. I was determined to.'

> 'Did what I could but not effectively.'

Some people spoke of coping after a fashion, but the following quotations typify the sorts of answers received from clients in this group:

> 'I didn't go out, got on with it, you have to, don't you, the best way you can.'

> 'Managed, but it was bad. People did not realise I was partially sighted.'

For those patients who are losing sight gradually and where deterioration in the early stages may be minimal and may allow them to adjust gradually over a period of time, this interim waiting time assumes less significance. It is for those patients who have suffered traumatic loss that any unnecessary delay may cause the greatest hardship and anguish. As summarised in some of the reflections from this group, several spoke of injuring themselves during this waiting period, with one lady talking of burning and scalding herself on the cooker and of being unsure of how to negotiate domestic chores with failing eyesight. Other clients spoke of burning themselves and their families. Early identification of those most in need of particular assistance, such as mobility training and emergency daily living skills, could forestall such serious consequences:

> 'I scalded myself once and set myself alight while cooking, so now I go into a "home" every day for my main meal.'

> (Female, blind, age 65–79.)

The elderly are potentially a very vulnerable and generally overlooked group. They often live alone and are socially isolated, are less likely to have the support of family and their own peer group is also likely to be elderly and less able to offer assistance. Therefore, the elderly group in particular might benefit from early assessment and intervention from social service departments.

'I managed to burn and scald myself.'

(Male, blind, degenerative, age 65"79.)

What emerges from the evaluation of clients' coping abilities during this interim period is that whilst most coped adequately on a physical day to day basis, there were instances of patients being significantly at risk as a consequence of their failing visual capabilities. Such risks could be minimised or completely overcome by earlier assessment and intervention. For those individuals who have lost sight traumatically or totally, the need for assistance becomes urgent; and perhaps for the elderly population within the visually impaired group as a whole, early rehabilitation becomes that much more imperative, because loss of sight may be only one of mixed disabilities commonly associated with ageing.

Clients' perceptions of help most needed

Perhaps not surprisingly one of the commonest responses to this enquiry was that there was most concern about matters of practical daily living. Mobility, transport, coping around the home and kitchen were all high on the list. Clients also expressed anxiety concerning financial planning and felt that general help and advice was needed in this area. Several just spoke of needing practical help generally with things:

'Help around the kitchen.'

'Transport.'

'Advice how to get around the shop.'

'Getting around outside.'

'I needed help with money and finance.'

However, once again it was noted that replies from several people hinted at a level of emotional distress and dis- ease about their disability. A sense of wistfulness and yearning to have their sight back:

'What I needed was my sight, and a few more friends.'

'All I wanted was my sight back.'

'I was sitting and crying.'

The effects of social isolation and lack of confidence discussed earlier in this chapter was highlighted in the replies from two participants:

'I wanted to talk about how I felt. I was worried about getting around. I got a lot of confidence and help from mobility officer eventually though.'

(Male, aged 40.)

'I wanted help with coins, telephones, meeting other blind people and going out together, some sort of outdoor activity to expel the way I feel sometimes.'

(Female, partially sighted.)

One gentleman spoke of wanting to use the time usefully to enjoy things as he had once done, which hints at the need for underlying assistance in rebuilding his life style and self identity:

'A club where I could use my hands and meet other people.'

In Chapters 6 and 7 we explored a multi-faceted approach to assisting clients to adjust to visual impairment. Such an approach will consider emotional, psychological, intellectual, philosophical and social predisposition and re-sponses to loss, addressing the issue of how to rebuild anew a lifestyle on the basis of an altered identity. The counselling model explores family networks and social support systems, identifies personal strengths and deficits which the client can appropriately enhance or redress. A multi-dimensional approach has the advantage of offering practical assistance, rehabilitative training, and counselling which addresses every aspect of the affected individual's lifestyle.

A couple of the people interviewed stated they were not sure what help was available and were therefore not aware what particular help they realistically needed. Several people felt they did not need any particular help:

'I didn't think I felt in need of assistance.'

'I had no particular difficulties.'

Clients' perceptions of their needs and individual situation has to be of paramount importance; any evaluation of the care given has to start from the basic premise that clients are caught in a situation and know where their greatest difficulty lies. However, we are all familiar with the situation where the social worker may define a whole constellation of difficulties as requiring assistance which the clients themselves may not have consciously registered, or indeed be prepared to admit. There can be no truly effective intervention while clients and workers hold different views about what assistance might be required. Exploring what type of help and assistance might be required in the early days following registration provides an opportunity to clarify what help is needed in the short term, but equally promotes an alliance of worker and client to prognosticate for the long term planning of rehabilita-tion.

The types of help offered and perceived usefulness

In evaluating the usefulness and effectiveness of assistance offered, it is useful to bear in mind that only just under two-thirds of the interviewed group had been visited by either a technical officer for the blind or a generic social worker. The remainder of the group could either not remember or gave no answer about who had visited them. Just under a third, 33 people, waited up to six months for a visit from the local social services department. Four unfortunate clients claimed they had to wait one year, with one further person stating he was not visited at all. Some also claimed that only after telephoning or chasing up their social service department were they visited. Such delays therefore might have some impact on clients' evaluation of usefulness of services received when eventually offered. There was a tendency for the blind to view the services that were offered most positively than did the partially sighted, 25 (45%) of blind clients defined the services offered as very useful, as against 13 (31%) of the partially sighted group, with 18 defining assistance offered as useful in the blind group, as against nine in the partially sighted group. Whilst no firm conclusions can be drawn from such tendencies, they might suggest that services have an inherent bias in the range of assistance offered towards those individuals who have little or no sight. However, it would also mean that the greater degree of deterioration, the more such assistance is needed and therefore the more it is appreciated and positively commented upon. For example, if a client has a small amount of residual vision then they might not be quite so dependent on braille literacy skills as a blind client. It was also noted that of the 22 who felt that the assistance offered was not very useful, 17 fell within the partially sighted group.

Commensurate with clients' perceptions about where their greatest difficulty lay in coping with visual impairment, a large section of the group reported that the help they were offered had been centred around practical assistance—mobility training and aids to daily living. Whilst most spoke warmly and positively about the help they had been offered, their verbatim comments displayed a wide variation of both the range and intensity of assistance provided even within the same borough. For example:

'Talking book, TV concession, Rehab Group, mobility, white stick, extra lighting and occupational items.'

'No help. Stick offered. I got some financial grant from the DHSS.'

Such a disparity of service may be explained by some clients having been seen by a specialist worker and others visited by a generic social worker.

Although the majority of them itemized talking books, talking newspapers, marked cookers, mobility training, and braille classes as being amongst the most useful services offered, there was a sense from some group members of compliance and resignation about whatever assistance they were offered. The impression was conveyed that they would be unlikely to request additional services and rehabilitation training despite feeling dissatisfied about the sort of assistance received:

> 'Didn't offer much, day centre and talking books, that is all.'

> 'Came and gave me a stick and a wireless, nothing more.'

It was also noticed that where technical officers or specialist workers had been involved, the range of services provided and access to rehabilitation and orientation training tended to be greatest. However, perhaps surprisingly, even when it appeared that the workers had provided a comprehensive range of services (as in the following quote) the inference was that the help provided could have gone further:

> 'The technical officer refreshed my braille skills, she brought me a braille typewriter, books, paper, a clock, writing frame, something to sort out coins in, only a few facilities.'

This might indicate that any amount of help would never be enough to meeting clients' internal psychic needs. It was noted that for others counselling was listed amongst the help provided—an opportunity to talk about how they felt, especially in relation to making practical adjustments to their lifestyle and routine:

> 'Practical help, especially in the kitchen, clubs, mobility, but also talking about how I felt using these things.'

Who most helped with talking through feelings about loss of sight

Having established that just under a third of the total group (33%) would have welcomed counselling and emotional help both at the time of registration and later, one may speculate about whether social workers and other involved carers are meeting this apparent need. We asked the clients to define who they felt had helped them most through their feelings about their loss of sight. Just under a quarter, 25 people, felt they had been most helped by their family:

> 'My sister, though I am a very private person normally.'

> 'My brother and sister-in-law, though at the time I thought I was going to die.'

> 'My wife helped me before she died.'

It is not surprising that family members appeared to play a significant part in helping the affected individuals to work through their feelings about loss of sight, as they are generally more accessible, sharing the day to day experience with the disabled person. As has been stressed earlier in this book, not every disabled person requires or wants counselling, and family members may unconsciously assume the role of informal counsellor and befriender, helping the visually impaired person to ventilate and off-load a whole range of feelings about loss of sight. However, the family as a whole and individually will have their own feelings and thoughts about what has happened to their loved one. Guilt and regret are generally common reactions because they feel unable to foresee or prevent the illness or disability. Thus the family may not be in a good position to offer emotional support, needing rather an opportunity to explore their own responses to the situation. This was summarised by one young lady:

> 'I can't really say anyone helped. My family were too emotionally involved themselves. If speaking about practically "physically" I would say my relatives helped there.'

Others spoke of friends or neighbours or, in some cases, church members offering quite a lot of emotional support. One lady spoke of faith in God being her mainstay of support:

> 'I put my faith in God. That kept me going.'

A major life event such as this may evoke a crisis of faith, undermining previously held belief. It is not uncommon, especially where there has been religious conviction, for initial fantasies concerning God's judgment for some perceived misdemeanor to abound—will the disability be viewed as divine retribution, for example, 'What have I done to deserve this?'

The most striking finding at this point was that the remainder of the group asserted that nobody had helped them at all. Two felt that it was a private battle which had to be fought alone:

> 'On my own. I suppose best left alone. I watched disabled sports on TV and there were blind people running and going over hurdles. It really made me think. I thought if they can do it, so can you, fight it, fight it, don't give in.'

> 'It's something you have to do on your own.'

> 'Nobody. I don't think or talk about it. My only hope is that I will not actually go blind before I die.'

It was noted that not one person interviewed cited a social worker as having helped them to talk through their feelings about loss of sight. This could, however, be due to the fact that skilled social workers may help clients talk about their feelings whilst ostensibly focusing on another task, such as mobility training or braille literacy skills. Furthermore, the client might have a specific stereotype of the worker in mind, seeing their role mainly as helping them to overcome the practical challenges of daily living, and therefore not perceiving their social worker in the role of counsellor. It has been said 'the best and most effective therapy and counselling is one where the patient is not aware that they have been counselled'. Furthermore, many clients may not like to admit to themselves retrospectively that they required counselling and emotional support; therefore they may edit this insight from their recollections and this may colour their comments about the emotional help and counselling received. It seemed there was a tendency to over—praise the practical help given by social workers. The reason for this seemed uncertain.

Historically, and until relatively recently, the training, orientation and mandate of specialist workers has been to provide practical rehabilitation training. The segregation of specific tasks within the rehabilitation field, with mobility officers, home teachers for the blind and, more recently, technical officers for the blind undertaking separate tasks may have had some influence on this process. The inexperienced generic or specialist worker might have their own misgivings about delving too deeply into the clients' psychological or emotional responses. Such reluctance may not be consciously acknowledged, but will be manifest through the workers looking no more deeply than the presenting problem; whether it is to supply a white stick or to arrange residential rehabilitation training. The limitations of time, coupled with the amount of material needed to be covered in the social work training curriculum, cannot, with the best will in the world, equip the new worker to have in-depth insights either into his own motivation for particular modes of intervention or equip him with all the necessary skills for counselling potentially distressed individuals. It is appropriate that workers should be able to acknowledge the limitations of their own experience and skills and to recognise that there is a fine line between 'going where angels fear to tread' and facilitating a client to share painful feelings which he might be shielding from the family. As the social worker may be the only independent person to discuss concerns with, it is regrettable that workers emotionally defend themselves to avoid the pain and distress a patient may call forth, and in so doing lose the opportunity to help the client develop a stronger sense of self and social skills. Good training and supervision can provide the social worker with sufficient confidence, skill and experience to tolerate his or her client's distress and thus potentially to work more humanely and effectively with them. It is to be hoped that the new syllabus to be pioneered for rehabilitation workers, whose ethos will be to combine the activities of these traditionally separate professional roles, may serve to balance these concerns.

Did rehabilitation services change consumers' perceptions about visual impairment?

Overall there was a general impression that where the full range of rehabilitation services had been made available to clients this had, at some level, changed their perception of visual impairment and the way they felt about loss of sight. There was also a feeling of reassurance in knowing there was someone whom they could contact in times of trouble:

'Nice to have someone I can ring. I had a letter after social worker's visit saying I could ring if I needed help. That is very reassuring to know.'

'Yes, there is someone who cares.'

Others, not surprisingly, spoke of increased confidence following mobility training and other rehabilitative services:

'Mobility training was very helpful. I got my confidence back.'

'Yes, more confident about getting about.'

In one particular instance it appeared that the social worker had directly facilitated an alternative philosophy for the client, and opened up new avenues of thinking about her response to the disability:

'The social worker said you must let people help you, be strong about it, but let them give it, do not go into a shell. This helped me a lot. I started to think about it.'

Whilst several clients spoke positively about the range of rehabilitation services offered, training and new skills had not affected the way they felt about visual impairment:

'No, I still feel the same way about my loss of sight. The skills I learnt were a great help but nothing could change the way I feel.'

'No, I was resigned to all that. Nothing could help the way I felt.'

This perhaps highlights the need for assistance which specifically address the client's feelings about loss. Whilst it is fair to say that clients' evaluation of social services provision was in the main positive and appreciative, there was a prevailing sense of something missing. Practical help had been appreciated but somehow the benefits of increased mobility and confidence had not been the panacea for their difficulties and the help offered had not gone as far as it might. This was emphasized from the account of those asked how they saw the future now, after practical help and rehabilitation had been offered by their respective social services departments. It was evident from the majority of replies that many clients were still unable to plan for the future, showing tendency to live from day to day and suggesting a level of resigned depression. The following quotes are fairly typical of those in this sub group:

'I live from week to week.'

'Day by day as it comes.'

'Oh, just getting by the best way I can.'

'I take one day at a time.'

It was noted with concern that the remaining clients in this group seemed to have little that was positive to hold onto for the future, and their comments suggested a level of despair:

'I have no future.'

'It doesn't seem all that bright to me.'

'Not very bright.'

'Don't see it, no future.'

'I sometimes worry. All my brothers and sisters are back in Sri Lanka. What if I am knocked over in the street and get crippled as well.'

'I really try not to think about it. At times I do, passing thoughts, but I don't dwell on it.'

'I see the future the same as I did before. I wait until God comes and fetches me.'

(Female, blind, degenerative, 80 plus.)

There can be many reasons why people feel despairing, uncertain or resigned about the future. For those reaching the twilight of their life, it is inevitable and to some extent appropriate that their thoughts will naturally turn to the past rather than the future. As one gentleman put it 'preparing oneself for the inevitable', and visual impairment may be viewed as part of a larger tapestry of life. Notwithstanding the above, a significant number of those who expressed feelings of resignation and hopelessness for the future were in their middle years, where such a response should not be glibly accepted as unavoidable. I would suggest that these responses are inappropriate and may be considered to be out of character for the affected individual's previous attitudes and philosophy before loss of sight and, as such, might demonstrate that the individual would benefit from a level of counselling formulating an altered lifestyle, learning to effectively accept what cannot be changed but equally important to change what can be changed. (see Table 8.1).

Summary

Whilst it is indicated that the majority of the disabled who were interviewed coped reasonably well in the interim period between registration at the hospital and a visit from the local social services department, it was noted with concern that several individuals, particularly the elderly, who were suffering severe or traumatic sight loss were potentially left at serious risk. There were incidents of scalding and burning whilst undertaking domestic chores at home. It was suggested that such mishaps could have been avoided with earlier assessment and intervention.

Table 8.1. Evaluation of rehabilitation

Evaluation of rehabilitation	Origin of Loss			
	Blind		Partially Sighted	
Very useful	25	44%	14	31%
Useful	18	31%	9	20%
Not very useful	5	7%	6	13%
Don't know	4	6%	2	6%
Can't remember	1	2%	0	
No answer	7	10%	13	30%
Total	60	100%	44	100%

The 'consumer' evaluation suggested that practical help from social services such as mobility training, aids to daily living and general advice about finance and benefits were issues of primary concern to most people. Equally, several spoke of a level of emotional distress and dis-ease about their disability. Many spoke of social isolation and lack of confidence being an early consequence of deteriorating vision as something with which they would have appreciated assistance.

It appeared that specialist workers were more likely to offer a greater range and variety of rehabilitation skills than their generic counterparts, which suggests the need for in- service training for generic social workers in order to familiarize them with the implications of visual impairment and to develop specific skills and expertise in this area. However, there was a sense from one or two clients that no amount of practical rehabilitation would be enough to meet their unique practical and emotional needs for assistance.

Whilst one or two listed counselling amongst the help provided, ident-ifying an opportunity to talk about how they felt, this was principally in relation to making practical adjustments to their lifestyle and routine. Not surprisingly, family and friends were among the main groups identified as being available to help the impaired person work through their feelings about loss of sight. Whilst the informal and necessary support of kith and kin should be acknowledged and welcomed, it was somewhat disquieting that not one person in the group defined their specialist worker or social worker as being directly responsible for helping them to work through their feelings. One of the most striking features of this enquiry was that a great proportion of those interviewed asserted that no one had helped them to talk about their feelings, and that they were left alone to cope with the necessary changes.

Encouragingly, there was a feeling from some clients that, broadly speak-ing, the intervention of rehabilitative services had impinged upon and changed their perceptions about visual impairment and the way they felt about the loss of sight. The most notable improvements were an increase in confidence and assertiveness, feeling reassured that there was a professional person they could turn to in times of trouble. One lady identified her social worker as being directly responsible for facilitating an altered philosophy in relation to her disability. Several in the group, although positively commenting on the range of rehabilitation services offered, qualified their praise by saying that training and new skills had not in themselves affected the way they felt about visual impairment, and that they continued to experience difficulty in the area of emotional adjustment.

Whilst it is fair to say that clients' evaluation of social services provision was in the main positive and appreciative, there was a prevailing sense of something missing. Such feelings were given weight by the number of people who even after rehabilitation had a bleak and pessimistic view of the future; unable to plan, living from day to day. It is suggested that such a response denotes underlying chronic depression and inability to come to terms with the reality of visual impairment and changed circumstances. It would appear that an interventional bias in favour of counselling and working in conjunction with practical rehabilitation might facilitate a more complete psycho-social tolerance for clients, which might facilitate practical rehabilitation to be taken up and used more effectively in consequence.

Recommendations

1. Earlier identification of those most in need; assessment and intervention should minimize the level of risk to visually impaired clients in the early phase of visual deterioration.

2. There is a need for structured in-service training for generic social workers on specific aspects of disability including a basic understanding of the implications of visual impairment.

3. The over 70s or those losing sight traumatically or who have lost a substantial degree of useful vision might benefit from targeted short-term crisis intervention whilst awaiting long-term rehabilitation training.

4. The ethos and philosophy of the social work profession generally might benefit from a more tolerant and facilitating view of the social worker's own needs in relation to working with acutely distressed individuals. Social workers might benefit from encouragement to consider their own defensive responses, the limitations of skill and experience, and to develop greater confidence and ability in intervention at varying levels with their clients.

Chapter 9

Arriving and Feeling Comfortable
The Question of Adjustment

Introduction

Throughout this book those factors which go to make up the visually impaired person's career in disability have been considered. In charting patients' motivation to seek assistance with initial sight difficulties, it has been a concern to explore the manner in which they were dealt with by their general practitioner and ophthalmic out-patient departments. One of the prime questions raised by this study is to consider in what ways the explanation of diagnosis and prognosis may help or hinder the patient's long term adjustment to his or her visual impairment. The concept of adjustment is a nebulous and often abused phrase. In consequence its meaning will vary from individual to individual. As a starting point, the definition given by the Concise Oxford Dictionary will suffice: namely, 'to adjust (adjustment) is to arrange, put in order, or harmonise'. This definition of adjustment may be in its broadest sense commonly acceptable to most people, and as such provides a working definition. In order to clarify what is meant by normal or healthy adjustment we have also drawn upon widely based theoretical models of grief and bereavement influenced by Murray-Parkes (1970), Pincus (1976) and others who speak of the stages of mourning and grief in working towards the resolution and acceptance of the reality of loss, culminating in the reinstatement of psychological equilibrium. We have also explored psychological research studies relating to visual impairment and blindness. Cholden (1958) defines three stages in the psychological response to loss of sight:

1) *Depersonalization*, which induces in the disabled person a short period of immobility, blankness or muteness. It is suggested that such a response is the ego's defence against bombardment of intolerable, overwhelming painful effect.

2) *Depression*, which involves mourning for lost sight. 'The death of the sighted person in order to be reborn as blind.' It has been noted by Fitzgerald (1970) and others, also in this study, that denial of the permanency of loss inhibits progression to the final stage in the process of adjustment, that of

3) *Recovery*, which usually results in the development of an alternative, tolerable lifestyle.

Certain pathological reactions which become entrenched, such as chronic dependency, prolonged depression and inappropriate undue idealization of other visually impaired people, have been considered. Cholden's postulated healthy recovery stage is seen to include the onset of problem-solving connected to visual impairment. Accompanying this response there is usually an overall resignation towards the fact that blindness is a handicap. From this point forward some progression is usually achieved. Such conclusions suggest that healthy adjustment to loss of sight is attained when the third phase is reached. A client once unwittingly defined this subtle change by saying she knew she could cope with her disability 'now' because she realized for the first time, in a long time, that she actually felt comfortable with herself. Theoretically, being able to accept that one is handicapped by reason of visual defect yet nevertheless tolerating this reality and retaining an overall sense of well being, seems to indicate the positive construction of adjustment. Notions of healthy adjustment were elaborated in the case of Mary, and to some extent with Lottie's situation, as presented in Chapter 7.

It would seem that for each individual there are two main levels of adjustment, both of which have to be achieved in order that a total and harmonious resolution is attained. The first level relates to overall practical adjustment. The results from this study suggest that practical adjustment is easier to achieve to an agreed level of satisfaction, and to maintain without major fluctuations. There was far less evidence of practical deterioration when compared with psychological and emotional responses. We all have to make compromises in our daily lives, but in responding to the onset of visual impairment many more compromises, both practical and psychological, may be necessary. Such compromise was emphasised by one woman when reflecting on the way she had adjusted to her loss of sight:

> 'I can still make tea. I have problems but at a pinch I can still do things. I "control" the cooking but do not actually do it myself.'

In Chapter 6 we explored the view that it is possible to adjust superficially to the changes wrought by loss of sight, whilst still struggling with less obvious psychological difficulties. An individual may adjust in part only, both psychologically and practically, which for the particular person affected may be the optimum level of adjustment, i.e. sufficient to meet specific needs. It is presumptuous to sit in judgment about what constitutes total or complete adjustment, even if such a thing were possible to measure. Professional assessment and criteria of adjustment may be very different from the expectations, aspirations and beliefs of patients. As one gentleman suggested:

> 'I have adjusted and accepted this situation, but not fully. I have to cope with it because there is nothing else to do.'

Another lady gave an example of the contrasts in her response:

> 'I have mentally adjusted but am frustrated when it takes me an hour to do something that would normally take a few minutes, then I feel sorry for myself.'

Such a response seems understandable and natural. We have to constantly consider the balance in distinguishing what is a healthy anticipated response and what might be a pathological reaction, both generally and in specific relationship to individual circumstances. If patients feel there is something out of character or not right for them, then this should be addressed. It may be that all that is needed is reassurance and help with understanding why they are feeling or reacting in a particular way. On the other hand, their response may constitute some level of unhelpful adjustment for them personally. In tandem with the personality assessment explored in the preceding chapter, in which a more objective analysis of overall reactions and potential adjustment to loss of sight was attempted, the study has sought the patients' evaluation of adjustment. They were asked to rate how they felt they had adjusted overall (see Table 9).

Table 9.1. Adjustment by extent of sight loss

Levels of adjustment	Blind No.	%	P/S No.	%	Total numbers	Total Percentages
Not at all	1	2	2	5	3	100
Moderately	29	52	19	45	48	100
Very well	22	37	15	33	37	100
No answer	7	9	9	17	16	100
Total	59	100	45	100	104	100

Taking into account the size differential between the blind and partially sighted groups, it would appear that registered blind people fared marginally better in terms of adjustment than the partially sighted. A slightly higher proportion of blind patients reported that they had adjusted either moderately or very well. From the total group, three stated that they had not adjusted at all, and it was noted that two of these were partially sighted. Whilst no firm conclusions can be drawn from these findings, these responses might support the view that the greater the deterioration, paradoxically the easier it is to adjust. Several factors may account for this. Greenblatt (1986) found in her study, which was primarily concerned with the interaction between ophthalmologists and their patients, that there was a trend for those patients with less severe impairments 'to receive less in the way of referrals or services from ophthalmologists' (6.a). To date, most studies on visual impairment have concentrated almost exclusively on blindness and its effects. This study recommends that further investigation into the responses and adjustment pattern of the partially sighted would prove fruitful.

Although those who felt they had not adjusted at all were in a small minority, their comments seem to suggest difficulty with both practical and emotional adjustment:

'I am afflicted, in almighty God's hands. Adjusted? Not at all!'

(Male, partially sighted, degenerative, age 40–64).

'I have not come to terms with it (sight loss). I feel as terrible. I would do anything to have it back. I get very bad tempered but I have to trust in God, haven't I? I haven't had a very pleasant life.'

(Female, partially sighted, age 80+).

This study also set out to consider whether age or gender had a significant impact on levels of adjustment. The three patients who claimed not to have adjusted at all fell into each of the three age bands, ranging from 64 years to 80+. This might suggest that age is not necessarily a contributory factor determining inability to adjust. For the group who felt that they had moderately adjusted, once again the age distribution was fairly evenly spread throughout the age bands. However, it was noted that in the middle age bands particularly, 65–79 years of age, a slightly higher number felt they had adjusted well; 18 as against 16 in the 80+ group. Gender did not appear to be a factor affecting the degree of adjustment obtained.

It is encouraging that the majority of those interviewed in both the partially sighted and blind groups felt they had adjusted either moderately or very well. This says much for individual courage and adaptability, and reflects positively on rehabilitation services. For those people who felt that they had adjusted moderately, a mixture of both optimism tinged with resignation was displayed:

'I can't read letters or do things that I would like to do around the house. There are no shortage of family and friends to do this, and I am beyond the stage that I don't like asking.'

(Male, blind, degenerative, age 40–60).

'I have stopped knitting. A few little things I can no longer do around the home, but nothing very much. I believe in God and He helps me over most of my problems.'

One lady attributed her moderate adjustment to 'having a place for everything.' Other people identified sharing the change with family as being supportive and aiding adjustment. It was suggested by one lady that just by accepting everything helped adjustment. Another confidently asserted that mental attitude had a lot to do with her adjustment:

'It has a lot to do with your mind. If your mind is active you can see and cope better.'

(Female, blind, degenerative, age 65–79).

Several in this moderate group appeared to shrug off the impact of their disability, with many asserting that it had little effect on their overall lifestyle and that little had changed because of visual impairment:

'It has not changed my life. I can still do the same things.'

'Everything takes longer, but I do everything very carefully. I enjoy all the things that I can do.'

One gentleman summed up the fairly typical feeling of others in this group when he said: 'I just cope some days better than others'. As might be expected, even where patients felt that they had adjusted well there was still a sense of unfinished business and a working through requirement:

'I still have feelings to sort out. I keep having setbacks, three heart attacks in two years!'

Another lady was even more specific about residual feelings concerning her disability:

'I still feel resentful that I am blind, that I have to walk with a cane or a guide dog and depend on other people, not being able to live a normal life as I would like.'

(Female, blind, degenerative, age 20–39).

One gentleman showed that one might have come generally to terms with loss of sight but still experience intense emotional reactions:

'I have come to terms with it, only sometimes I desperately want to be able to see something. Recently I saw a German film. My German was not good enough to understand the plot. It would have helped, for example, to see what was happening.'

Despite the results of this study that there appears to be greater difficulty with issues of intellectual and psychological resolution, nevertheless it is heartening that the majority of the group felt they had achieved a reasonable level of adjustment.

Of the 37 people in the group who felt that they had adjusted very well, it was noted that several of these had managed to use their experience and the potential crisis of change to positive advantage. The term 'grief to growth', which implies that out of adversity and sorrow can come personal growth and new insight, giving realization of hitherto unknown qualities, seemed to have relevance for some in the group:

'It doesn't bother me too much. I have come to terms with it. I do a lot of other things now which I never had the time for before, i.e. learning German and Italian, swimming, etc.'

'I can use my hands better now.'

> 'I thought my lifestyle would change. I have a lot less money but I have so much more time to do all the things I have always wanted to do.'

One gentleman responded to the question 'In what ways have you adjusted to your loss of sight?' cryptically with:

> 'I have adjusted all ways. I have learned to make use of "outer vision". I have survived.'

The majority who asserted that they had adjusted either moderately or very well repeatedly displayed a level of resignation or stoicism in relation to visual deterioration. To consider that they were in any sense making the best of a bad job does their courage and determination an injustice. Underlying the statements from these people was the feeling they had come to tolerate the limitations of their disability whilst retaining the highest possible level of independence and dignity:

> 'I have tried to go out walking on my own. I try to do the best I can always.'

> 'I am thankful for what I can see and do. Loss of vision is not my main problem.'

> 'I just take changes as they come.'

Whilst most people were able to hold onto their affirmation that they were either adjusting or had come through the most turbulent phases, it was equally apparent, and not surprising, that thoughts and questions about the future were uppermost in their minds and fairly prevalent amongst the group. Several feared further sight deterioration or becoming increasingly helpless and dependent:

> 'I have worries about changes sight loss will bring.'

> 'I worry about going totally blind'.

> 'Frightened in case my sight gets worse and I end up blind and useless.'

Conclusion

The results from this study suggest that, contrary to former belief, psychological and emotional adjustment appear to pose greater difficulty for visually impaired people than practical adjustment. Clients' evaluation of their achievements in connection with adjustment generally suggest, however, a more positive picture. There seems little doubt from the information collected in this study, that greater emphasis needs to be placed on counselling and psychological help for visually impaired people. This is particularly important during diagnostic/prognostic sessions with patients and especially at the time of registration.

The study has considered the pressures and restraints placed upon medical and nursing personnel in busy ophthalmic out-patients departments and general practitioner services. We have considered how utilizing the skills of medical social workers, specialist rehabilitation workers or trained counsellors to work alongside ophthalmologists and general practitioners might help to share the burden of breaking bad news to patients, providing them with an initial early opportunity to ventilate feelings and raise questions, provide information, identify patients most in need of crisis intervention, and make appropriate referrals for on- going assistance. It was postulated that the instigation of a multi-disciplinary team approach and counselling service might alleviate some of the delays which appeared to have arisen throughout the process of registration. An outline model of such a counselling service was presented along with case material, incorporating specific examples of alternative responses to particular problems posed by patients at various stages in their career of disability, such as suicidal tendency or denial.

Throughout this book the endeavour has been to present a comprehensive view of the potential for both positive personal development and growth out of crisis and for realistically exploring patients' vulnerability during the phase of loss of sight. Other than Fitzgerald's work in this country, relatively little research has been done into the difficult and subtle area of psychological response and adjustment. It will be remembered that one of the aims of this study was to address this omission, whilst valuing the personal experiences of the disabled consumer group. The study sought to combine both theoretical perspectives with clinical experience and consumer views. The aim was to elucidate and further discuss how we as professionals can improve the service we offer to visually impaired people. To listen to what patients have to tell us and to react realistically and sensitively. Such a facilitating response must ultimately be the overriding value of this type of study.

The people who took part in this survey co-operated fully in a courageous manner with a searching and sensitive interview. Many said their motivation for this was to know that they had in some way contributed to help other people who will follow after them and who may, in consequence, be dealt with differently and more appropriately.

It is hoped that any merit this study may contain will encourage individual professionals to reflect on their practice, attitudes and abilities. It has not been intended as a criticism of any particular discipline, but rather as encouragement to evaluation practice and constructively to consider how shortfalls may be avoided.

This book will conclude with a summary of recommendations drawn from the text.

Major Recommendations

General practitioner and ophthalmology health care services

1. More time needs to be allocated to general practitioners and consultant ophthalmologists to talk through with the clients the implications of diagnosis and prognosis. Patients need to be prepared both emotionally and practically for the onset of visual impairment.
2. Additional follow-up appointments need to be available for recapitulation and disclosure, one or two weeks after the initial diagnosis or prognosis has been given.
3. The instigation of a 'key worker' approach in clinics would increase the likelihood of consistent information being given to patients and facilitate rapport and good communications.
4. There needs to be a shift of emphasis in the selection and training of doctors and ophthalmologists—the training curriculum of medical schools would benefit from a greater awareness of counselling and communication skills.
5. Patient and staff ratios need to be re- evaluated in the light of current centralisation.

The registration process

6. The study concludes that the process of registration itself comes too late in the day for some patients who at the time of registration have lost a significant amount of vision. The study recommends that the entitlement of assistance and services should not be dependent upon the process of registration. It is recommended that emphasis be placed on the importance of facilitating early registration.
7. Rehabilitation training and assistance from social service departments should be made available both pre- and post-registration.
8. The voluntary nature of registration should be stressed to the affected individuals and their families at every stage of the registration process.
9. The involvement of a specialist social worker working with the consultant ophthalmologist from specialist registration clinics would provide early assessment and prioritization of those most in need of practical and emotional assistance.
10. Greater collaboration between hospital based consultant ophthalmologists and area social workers would promote the likelihood that no patients would leave hospital unaware that they have been registered and would facilitate early assistance, and would override bureaucratic procedures.
11. Additional administrative support in hospital based services might facilitate early completion of BD8 forms.
12. Further comparative research of clients who have received prophylactic assistance prior to registration and those experiencing delayed assistance might prove fruitful.
13. Earlier identification of those most in need; assessment and intervention should minimize the level of risk to visually impaired clients in the early phase of visual deterioration.

14. There is a need for structured in-service training for general social workers on specific aspects of disability including a basic understanding of the implications of visual impairment, registration and rehabilitative interventions.

15. The over 70s those losing sight traumatically or those who have lost a substantial degree of useful vision might benefit from targeted short-term crisis intervention whilst awaiting long-term rehabilitation training.

16. The ethos and philosophy of social work and caring professions generally might benefit from a more tolerant and facilitating view of their own needs in relation to working with acutely distressed individuals. Such workers might benefit from encouragement to consider their own defensive responses, the limitations of skill and experience, and to develop greater confidence and ability in intervention at varying levels with their clients.

Counselling services

17. Counselling may be a valuable precursor to rehabilitation thereby potentially increasing the likelihood of effective and practical intervention.

18. The study concludes that rehabilitation assistance and counselling (where provided) offered by social service departments should not be contingent on the client being registered or suitable for registration as visually impaired (partially sighted or blind).

19. Post qualification specific and general study in counselling techniques should be more widely available, possibly on the basis of in-service training.

20. The collaboration of all professionals involved in the care of the visually impaired would have healthy beneficial ripple effects for the client group as they move through the system.

21. The instigation of a structured multi- disciplinary counselling service would provide a cross fertilization of experience and philosophy increasing the likelihood of healthy all-round adjustment.

22. The philosophy underlying resource allocation should be enriched by concern with meeting 'internal' needs and concerns with the emphasis shifting away from mainly quantifiable 'external' and visible provision and activity.

23. The study recommends that further investigation into the responses and adjustment pattern of the partially sighted may prove fruitful.

Appendix

INTERVIEW FORMAT

RESEARCH INTO THE RESPONSES, NEEDS AND SERVICES OFFERED TO NEWLY REGISTERED VISUALLY IMPAIRED PATIENTS

BOROUGH .... WHEN REGISTERED ....day ....month ....year

HOSPITAL ....

GENDER ....Male ....Female   ORIGIN OF SIGHT LOSS:

AGE   ....   Degenerative   .....   Blind   .....

    20–39   40–64   65–79   80+   Trauma   .....   P/Sighted   .....

ENGLISH FIRST LANGUAGE: .OTHER DISABILITIES:

    Yes   .....   No   .....   Hearing Impaired: Yes   .....   No   .....

RELIGIOUS DENOMINATION—PRACTISING:

Church of England	.....	Others—Specify .....
Roman Catholic	.....	....
Muslim	.....	....
Hindu	.....	....

IN EMPLOYMENT NOW: LAST EXAMINATION BEFORE
                                 CERTIFICATION

    Yes   .....   No   .... day ....month ....year

SOCIAL/ECONOMIC CLASS: DATE OF CERTIFICATION OF BD8:

Professional/Clerical   .... day ....month ....year

Manual   .....   DATE BD8 RECEIVED IN SOCIAL

Skilled   .....   SERVICES:

UnSkilled   .... day ....month ....year

                                     DATE OF FIRST CONTACT FROM
                                     SOCIAL SERVICES:

                                     .... day ....month ....year

INTERVIEWERS NAME: ....Date ....

PART ONE—PRE-REGISTRATION

1) Did you suspect sight loss prior to diagnosis? Yes ..... No .....
2) What prompted you to seek medical help from your G.P? ....
....
....

PROMPT: When you visited your G.P. was it for any of the following reasons?
Please answer yes or no:

(a) I put off seeking medical advice, Yes ..... No ..... No answer .....
(b) I was afraid there was something seriously wrong with my sight,
Yes ..... No ..... No answer .....

3) PROMPT: When you visited your G.P. did you feel any of the
following:

(a) I felt my G.P. was sympathetic about my anxiety,
Yes ..... No ..... No answer .....
(b) I felt my G.P. understood my feelings about my difficulty in seeing,
Yes ..... No ..... No answer .....
(c) I was satisfied with the way my G.P. dealt with me at this time,
Yes ..... No ..... No answer .....
(d) I was entirely satisfied with the attention I received from my G.P.,
Yes ..... No ..... No answer .....
What else would you like to say about your G.P.'s response when you visited him?
....
....
....

4) Was he:
Sympathetic .....
Unsympathetic .....
Don't Know .....
Can't remember .....
5) Did he seem:
Interested .....
Disinterested .....
6) Can you remember how long it was between the time you saw your doctor and your hospital appointment?
Yes ..... No .....
Time: ....

PROMPT: And now I would like to talk about the time when you went to the hospital!

7) From the first time you saw a hospital doctor, how long did you have to wait before your eye condition was adequately explained to you?

First appointment	.....	Within six months	.....
Within a week	.....	Don't know	.....
Within one month	.....	Can't Remember	.....
Within three months	.....	Never Explained	.....

7a) Were you given the same information by the different doctors that you saw?
Yes ..... No ..... D.K./C.R. ..... No answer .....
8) How did the hospital doctor explain your eye condition? ....
....
....
Was the explanation understandable?
Yes ..... No ..... D.K./C.R. ..... No answer .....

9) Did you feel that you were given:
   Adequate information   .....
   Inadequate information   .....
   Don't know   .....
   Can't remember   .....
10) Did your doctor help you prepare for your loss of sight?
   Yes .....   No .....   D.K./C.R.   .....   No answer   .....
   If so, how ....
   ....
   ....

11) Did you feel the doctor had time to discuss any difficulties with you?
   Yes .....   No .....
12) In what ways were you able to prepare emotionally for loss of sight?
   ....
   ....
   ....

13) In what ways were you able to prepare practically for loss of sight? ....
   ....
   ....

14) What assistance did you feel you need at this time? ....
   ....
   ....

15) Overall, could this experience have been improved for you?
   Yes .....   No .....
   If so, how? ....
   ....
   ....
   ....
   ....
   ....
   ....
   ....
   ....

PART TWO—REGISTRATION AS BLIND/PARTIALLY SIGHTED

1) How long after diagnosis was registration discussed?
   First appointment   .....
   Within one month   .....
   Within three months   .....
   Within six months   .....
   Within one year   .....
   Was not discussed   .....
   Don't know   .....
   Can't remember   .....
2) Who first discussed registration as being blind/partially sighted with you?
   Hospital doctor   .....
   Nurse   .....
   Other—Specify ....
3) What did it mean to you to be registered as blind/partially sighted?
   ....
   ....
   ....

4) What advantages did you see in being registered? ....
   ....

5) What disadvantages did you see in being registered? ....
   ....

6) Before you lost your sight, what did you think about blind/partially sighted people?
   ....

7) What were some of your feelings when you were told you were to be registered as
   blind/partially sighted? ....
   ....
   ....
   ....

8) How did you see the future ? ....
   ....
   ....
   ....

9) Overall was discussion about registration:
   Adequate   .....
   Inadequate   .....
   Don't know   .....
   Can't remember   .....
10) Did you ever consider seeking a second opinion?
   Yes   .....   No   .....   D.K./C.R.   .....   No answer   .....
10b) Did you seek a second opinion?
   Yes   .....   No   .....   D.K./C.R.   .....   No answer   .....
11) How did you think your life would change?
   ....
   ....
   ....
   ....

HOLISTIC ASSESSMENT

PROMPT: Have you ever felt or feel any of the following? Please answer yes or no. Interviewer, after each question please ask the following questions and tick appropriate boxes in column.
(a) Did you feel this before your loss of sight?
(b) At the time you lost you sight?
(c) Now?

		A	B	C
1) I could not accept that it had happened to me	Y/N	.....	.....	.....
2) I was worried about the changes it would bring	Y/N	.....	.....	.....
3) I could not talk honestly about my worries and feelings	Y/N	.....	.....	.....
4) I felt vulnerable	Y/N	.....	.....	.....
5) I did not like myself	Y/N	.....	.....	.....
6) I tried not to think about it	Y/N	.....	.....	.....
7) I could not accept that I would never get my sight back	Y/N	.....	.....	.....
8) I did not expect this to happen at my age	Y/N	.....	.....	.....
9) I could not see any hope for the future	Y/N	.....	.....	.....
10) I felt that the meaning and purpose had gone out of my life	Y/N	.....	.....	.....
11) I wondered what I had done to deserve this	Y/N	.....	.....	.....
12) I asked myself 'why me?'	Y/N	.....	.....	.....
13) I felt it was unfair	Y/N	.....	.....	.....
14) It made my question my faith	Y/N	.....	.....	.....
15) It made me examine my philosophy of life	Y/N	.....	.....	.....
16) I thought of taking my own life	Y/N	.....	.....	.....
16a) I made a suicide attempt	Y/N	.....	.....	.....
17) I felt my world had crumbled	Y/N	.....	.....	.....
18) I felt as if I were no longer acceptable	Y/N	.....	.....	.....
19) I felt like a second class person	Y/N	.....	.....	.....
20) I was afraid people would reject me	Y/N	.....	.....	.....
21) I was afraid other people would pity me	Y/N	.....	.....	.....
22) I became ill	Y/N	.....	.....	.....
23) I had no energy	Y/N	.....	.....	.....
24) I never felt healthy	Y/N	.....	.....	.....
25) I found myself				
(a) drinking more	Y/N	.....	.....	.....
(b) smoking more	Y/N	.....	.....	.....
(c) taking sedatives	Y/N	.....	.....	.....
26) I felt worried most of the time	Y/N	.....	.....	.....
27) I felt there was no hope for the future	Y/N	.....	.....	.....
28) I felt I could have done more to prevent this loss of sight	Y/N	.....	.....	.....
29) I felt someone else was to blame	Y/N	.....	.....	.....
30) I was bitter about my loss of sight	Y/N	.....	.....	.....
31) I felt angry	Y/N	.....	.....	.....
32) I felt sad about what had happened to me	Y/N	.....	.....	.....
33) I was longing to be able to see again	Y/N	.....	.....	.....
34) I felt so alone in this experience	Y/N	.....	.....	.....
35) I felt no one could understand what I was going through	Y/N	.....	.....	.....
36) I felt as though I would never feel again	Y/N	.....	.....	.....
37) I had mixed feelings	Y/N	.....	.....	.....
38) I made promises that if I got my sight back I would do something in return	Y/N	.....	.....	.....
39) I often felt embarrassed	Y/N	.....	.....	.....
40) I tried to cover up the fact that I could not see	Y/N	.....	.....	.....
41) I felt ashamed about being blind/partially sighted	Y/N	.....	.....	.....
42) I felt I would never be attractive to anyone again	Y/N	.....	.....	.....
43) I was afraid that I would never have an intimate relationship with anyone again	Y/N	.....	.....	.....

44) I felt there was nothing to get up for   Y/N   ....
45) I felt there was nothing in the week to look forward to   Y/N   ....
46) I felt other people organised my life   Y/N   ....
47) I felt choice had been taken out of my hands   Y/N   ....
48) I felt nothing worse could ever happen to me   Y/N   ....
49) I had a lot of other worries and stresses on me   Y/N   ....
50) I was afraid I would go mad   Y/N   ....
51) I felt I could not cope with anything else   Y/N   ....
52) I did not know how to behave around other people   Y/N   ....
53) I was unsure what other people would expect of me   Y/N   ....
54) Other people expect me to have got used to my loss of
    sight by now   Y/N   ....
55) People expect me to be grateful   Y/N   ....
56) I feel people will not let me be myself   Y/N   ....
57) My relationships with my family have changed   Y/N   ....
   (a) For the better   Y/N   ....
   (b) For the worse   Y/N   ....
58) I feel other people try to overprotect me   Y/N   ....
59) I feel other people have no faith in me anymore   Y/N   ....
60) I feel that people talk down to me   Y/N   ....
61) My family don't expect as much of me as they do of
    other people   Y/N   ....
62) I find it more difficult to make friends now   Y/N   ....
63) I feel that I am not achieving my potential   Y/N   ....
64) I have difficulty in looking after the home   Y/N   ....
65) I have difficulty in taking care of myself   Y/N   ....
66) I worry about my financial situation   Y/N   ....
67) I have difficulty getting around on my own   Y/N   ....
68) I have problems with my accommodation   Y/N   ....
69) I have problems with my job/studies   Y/N   ....
70) I felt that what was offered did not suit my individual
    needs   Y/N   ....
71) Thinking about these questions has brought back
    painful memories for me   Y/N   ....

PART THREE—POST REGISTRATION/AFTER CARE

PROMPT: Now I would like to talk to you about what happened to you after registration!

1) After registration who visited you to talk about helping you with your sight problems?
   a) Technical officer for the blind
   b) Social Worker   .....
   c) Other—Specify ....
   How long after?
   Within one week   .....
   Within one month   .....
   Within three months   .....
   Within six months   .....
   Within one year   .....
   Can't remember   .....
   Not at all   .....
2) What help were you offered? ....
   ....
3) How useful were these services for you personally?
   Very useful   .....
   Useful   .....
   Not very useful   .....
   Don't know   .....
   Can't remember   .....
4) Did you feel that the help you were offered was:
   (a) Made for you personally   Yes ..... No .....
   (b) That you had to fit in with what was available   Yes ..... No .....
5) What help did you feel most in need of? ....
   ....
6) Did you receive it?
   Yes .....   No .....   Don't Know ......   Can't remember .....
7) How did you manage before help was provided? ....
   ....
   ....
   ....
8) How do you see the future now?
   ....
   ....
   ....
9) Looking back over your experience, what sense have you been able to make of your loss of sight?
   ....
   ....
   ....
10) Who most helped you to work through your feelings about loss of sight? ....
   ....
   ....
   ....

PART FOUR—CONCLUSIONS

1) Do you feel you have adjusted to your loss of vision?

Not at all .....
A little .....
Moderately .....
Very well .....

PROMPT: By adjustment I mean that you have learned to live with this change, that you have learned practical ways of coping with limited sight and that you are gradually feeling more at ease with yourself; that you have accepted that this situation cannot be changed.

2) In what ways have you adjusted to your loss of sight?

....
....
....
....

3) In what ways, if any, have you not come to terms with this change? What problems have you had? ....

....
....
....

4) Did the services you received change the way you felt about your loss of sight?

Yes ..... No ..... D.K./C.R. ..... No answer .....
If so, how? ....

....
....

5) Given that loss of vision affects one's overall situation, would it have helped you to talk to a skilled person about your feelings and the change that loss of sight have imposed on you and your family, and to explore new ways of coping? Would this have been helpful to you?

Yes ..... No ..... D.K./C.R. ..... No answer .....

PROMPT: Thank you very much for taking part in this interview, which I feel sure is going to be of assistance in helping us to improve the services we can offer to other people who have lost, or are losing, their sight. Please let me assure you that everything you have told me will be treated in the strictest confidence and that no note has been made of your name and address.
Thank you once again.

Bibliography

Adams, G.L., Pearlman, J.T. and Sloan, S.H. (1971) 'Guidelines For Psychiatric Referral Of Visually Handicapped Patients'. *American Journal of Ophthalmology* 3, 72–73.

Ash, D., Keegan, D.L. and Greenough, T. (1978a) 'Factors in Adjustment to Blindness'. *Canadian Journal of Ophthalmology* 13, 15–21.

Ash, D., Keegan, D.L. and Greenough, T. (1978b) 'Psychological and Social Adjustment to Blind Subjects and the 16PF'. *Canadian Journal of Ophthalmology* 34 (1).

British Assessment of Counselling (1988)

Calek, O. (1980) 'Acceptance of Vocation and Visual Disability in Blind and Partially Sighted Students'. *International Journal of Rehabilitation* 3.

Cholden, L.S. (1958) *A Psychiatrist Works With Blindness*. New York: American Foundation for the Blind.

Circular 4/55 Ministry of Health Appendices III and IV. *No statutory definition could be traced.

Conyers, M.C. (1986) 'Emotional and Practical Adjustment to Loss of Sight'. Interim paper. Published for the [ACTA] 25th International Congress of Ophthalmology.

Cullinan, T.R., (1977) 'The Epidemiology of Visual Disability: Studies of Visually Disabled People in the Community'. University of Kent, Health Services Research Unit Report No. 28.

DHSS Satistics (March 1986)

Diamond, B.L. and Ross, A. (1945) 'Emotional Adjustment of Newly Blind Soldiers'. *American Journal of Psychiatry.*

Donnelly, D. (1986) 'The Problems and Needs of the Newly Registered Blind'. Unpublished paper. Manchester Royal Infirmary.

Dunton (Junior), W.R. (1908) 'Mental State of the Blind'. *American Journal of Insanity* 65, 103-112.

Finestone and Gold (1959) *The role of the Opthalmologist in the Rehabilitation of Blind Patients*. New York: American Foundation for the Blind/The Seeing Eye.

Fitzgerald, R.G. (1970) 'Reactions to Blindness—A Systemic and Exploratory Study in Adults with Recent Loss of Sight'. Archives of General Psychiatry, 370–379.

Greenblatt, S.L. (1986) 'Ophthalmologist Interactions With Visually Impaired Patients'. unpublished.

Hall, L. (1982) 'Who Are Britain's Blind People?' *New Society*, 377–379.

Hicks, S. (1981) 'Relationship and Sexual Problems of the Visually Handicapped'—in Brechin, A., Liddiard, P. and Swain, J. *'Handicap in a Social World'* edited by Anne Brechin, Penny Liddiard and John Swain. Hodder & Stoughton/Open University.

Hoehn-Saric, H., et al. (1981) 'Single Case Study—Coping with Blindness'. *Journal of Nervous and Mental Disease* 169.

Lukoff, J. and Whitman, M. (1972) *Social Sources of Adjustment to Blindness.* Research Series No. 21. New York: American Foundation for the Blind.

Murray-Parkes, C.M., (1970) *Bereavement—A Study of Grief in Adult Life. Harmondsworth/Penguin.*

National Assistance Act 1948.

Oehler-Giarranta, J. and Fitzgerald, R.G. (1980) 'Group Therapy With Blind Diabetics'. *General Psychiatry* 37 (4) 463–467.

Ollendick, T.H., (1985) 'Fears in Visually Impaired and Normal Sighted Youth'. *Journal of Behaviour, Research and Therapy* 23.

Pincus, L. (1976) 'Death in the Family'. ???London???: Faber & Faber Limited.

Rakes, S.M. and Reid, W.H. (1982) 'Psychologic Management of Loss of Vision'. *Canadian Journal of Ophthalmology* 17 (4).

Schultz, P.J. (1979) *Reactions to Loss of Sight.* In Pearlman, J.L., Adams, G.L. and Sloan et al (eds) Psychiatric Problems in Ophthalmology, ccThomas, Springfield, I11, 38–67

Shaw, J. 'The Registration of Blind and Partially Sighted People'. (An appraisal of the scheme in a southern country in England.) Central Birmingham Health District.

Shaw, P. (1985) 'Local Authority Social Rehabilitation Services to Visually Handicapped People.' *RNIB Report 8* (13) 127.

Sainsbury, E. (1983) 'Client Studies and Social Policy' in Fisher, M. (ed) *Speaking of Clients* Social Service Monographs: Research into practice. PLACE????: Joint Unit for Social Service Research.

Thurme, L. and Murphree, O.D. (1961) 'Acceptance of the White Cane and Hope for Restoration of Sight in Blind Persons as an Indication of Adjustment.' *Journal of Clinical Psychology* 17.

Whittkower, E. and Davenport, R.C., (1946) 'War Blinded, Their Emotional Social and Occupational Situation'. *Journal of Medical Psychology.*

Index

Adaptation 24, 70

Adjustment 23–26, 30, 34, 47, 52, 63, 76, 77, 81, 86–89, 91, 95, 102, 107, 118–125, 127

After care 106

Anger 23, 42, 54, 66, 71, 72, 81, 89, 92, 98, 99

Anxiety 23, 24, 26, 29, 31, 35, 42, 53, 55, 66, 79, 80, 94, 98, 99–101, 109

Autonomy 101

Career in disability 14, 21, 28, 58, 68, 71, 74, 119

Case presentation 91, 95

Certification 62, 63

Clinic 11, 31, 38, 39, 42–44, 53, 62

Consultant 38, 43, 46, 49, 50, 53, 64, 65, 95, 126

Counselling 12–14, 16–20, 25, 26, 30, 42–44, 54, 59, 64, 67, 71, 72, 74–76, 79, 81, 84, 87–92, 94, 95, 97, 98, 100, 101–106, 110, 112–114, 116–118, 124–127

Decision 17, 87

Degenerative 20, 29, 33, 34, 36, 37, 39–42, 45, 53, 54, 56, 57, 58–60, 68–70, 109, 116, 122

Denial 11, 12, 16, 22–24, 29, 30, 50, 56, 58, 66, 67, 69–72, 77, 79, 81, 92, 93, 97, 98, 119, 125

Despair 53, 59, 66, 67, 74, 81, 89, 90, 99, 116

Deterioration 25, 28–30, 40, 45, 52, 58, 66, 76–81, 83, 85, 89, 101, 108, 111, 118, 120, 121, 124, 126

Diagnosis 12, 14, 21, 25, 26, 29, 34–40, 42–44, 46–49, 63, 81, 98, 119, 126

Disability 14, 20, 21, 23, 24, 28, 55, 58, 66–68, 71, 74, 75, 77, 82–84, 92, 93, 95, 98, 107, 109, 113, 115, 118, 119, 120, 123–125, 127

Disbelief 22, 30, 53, 92

Eyesight 42, 46, 48, 69, 100, 108

Family 16, 18, 23, 24, 28, 39, 45, 47, 51, 54, 64, 67, 75, 80, 84, 88, 90, 92, 93, 95, 97, 98, 100, 104, 107, 109, 110, 112–114, 117, 122

Form BD8 46, 47, 62, 106

Friends 22, 45, 51, 67, 77, 108, 109, 113, 117, 122

General Practitioner 28–33, 46, 75, 78, 104, 119, 125, 126

Handicap 15, 17, 20, 22–24, 28, 45, 46, 57, 71, 76, 87, 92, 94, 102, 103, 107, 120

Insight 13, 22, 35, 50, 67, 79, 91, 93, 95, 123

Investigation 12, 13, 16, 21, 22, 24, 47, 48, 50, 52, 64, 90, 107, 127

Key worker 38, 44, 126

Loss of sight 11, 14–17, 20–26, 28–30, 34, 37–40, 42, 43, 45, 47, 50–52, 54, 56, 58, 66–68, 71, 74–79, 81, 82, 83–86, 88–92, 95, 102, 104, 106, 107, 109, 112, 113–118, 120, 121, 123, 125

Management 11, 12, 20, 21, 25, 34, 38, 42–44, 100, 101, 107

Mourning 22, 23, 30, 39, 100, 119

Negative Denial 56, 58, 67, 71, 72, 79

Negative Feelings 15, 59, 67, 92, 98, 116

Ophthalmologist 23, 25, 26, 34, 38–40, 42–44, 46–53, 55, 62, 63, 64, 91, 126

Ophthalmology 11, 18, 34, 41, 48, 126

Pain 28, 66, 79, 80, 92, 97, 99, 100, 114

Physical illness 54, 64

Prognosis 12, 25, 26, 38, 39, 43, 44, 46, 48, 81, 119, 126

Puzzlement 66, 79, 80

Refusal 66, 81

Registration 11, 12, 14, 18–21, 26, 27, 34, 42, 45–65, 87, 88, 90, 91,

104, 106–108, 110, 112, 116, 124–127

Rehabilitation 12, 14, 16, 18, 19, 23–26, 30, 34, 35, 39, 46, 48, 51, 60, 62, 72, 75, 77, 81, 83, 84, 86–92, 94, 102, 103, 104, 106, 107, 109, 110, 112, 114–117, 118, 122, 125–127

Resignation 30, 56, 97, 98, 111, 116, 120, 122, 124

Resource allocation 12, 86, 87, 105, 127

Sedatives 79

Self Esteem 39, 67

Self identity 52, 92, 110

Service provision 13, 23, 46, 86, 99, 101

Sight 11–17, 20–34, 37–43, 45–47, 50–52, 54–58, 63, 64, 66, 67, 68–71, 74–86, 88–93, 95, 101, 102, 104, 106, 107, 108, 109, 111–125, 127

Smoking 79

Social Status 23, 45

Stigmatization 55, 67

Stoicism 30, 56, 108, 124

Suicide 14–16, 22, 54, 64, 67, 71, 74, 75, 97, 125

Support 12, 13, 18, 27, 38, 39, 51, 57, 58, 61, 62, 65, 79, 87, 88, 90, 97, 98, 101, 104, 106–110, 113, 114, 117, 121, 126

Technical officers 17, 18, 112, 114

Training 12–15, 17, 18, 27, 43, 44, 64, 66, 67, 77, 87, 89, 91, 92, 94, 95, 97, 101, 103, 104, 106, 108, 110, 111–115, 117, 118, 126, 127

Understanding 11, 13, 14, 22, 34, 37, 42, 48, 49, 68, 91, 99, 101, 104, 106, 107, 118, 121, 127

Worry 66, 68, 79, 80, 116, 124

Yearning 109

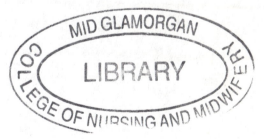